# MANUAL OF KINESIOLOGICAL TAPING

An epitome of kinesiology taping techniques

I0487747

FIRST
EDITION

## Dedications:

This book is dedicated to:

My idols Joginder Yadav sir and Ananda Jothi Chandrasekaran sir

My mother and father, Aruna and Ramesh Chand Jain

My wife Tanvi Jain

My brother Ayush Jain

My teachers and guides.

# PREFACE

Kinesiological taping methods can help in providing the physiotherapist a great tool to serve his patient with great result in conjunction to other therapeutic modalities. No treatment protocol can work without a proper assessment of the patients, the need of clinical reasoning with proper assessment tools are the basic necessity of the therapist. The use of kinesiology taping was started in Japan by Dr. Kenzo Kase, from there it has spread as the most effective taping technique to whole of the world. The kinesiology tapes can be used in almost all the fields of physiotherapy ranging from orthopedics to sports, to gynecology and much more.

This book is a reference text for the kinesiology taping therapists who are trained in the method of taping. The basic steps given in the book can make a practicing therapist to use taping technique innovatively to the subjects in different clinical conditions. The book is a researched based approach to the effect of kinesiology taping in different conditions, structure and functions of body.

The book is written with its associated institute, INSTITUTE OF KINESIOLOGY TAPING. IKT is entitled to use the content of the book as a training script only.

As kinesiological taping is an emerging field in India, there is great need of good therapists and researchers in this field. The book's content may be revised time to time with latest advancements and new researches.

**PIYUSH JAIN**

**INSTITUTE OF KINESIOLOGY TAPING**

**INDIA**

# CONTENTS

4. FASCIA AND LYMPHATIC CORRECTION

# CHAPTER 1

# INTRODUCTION

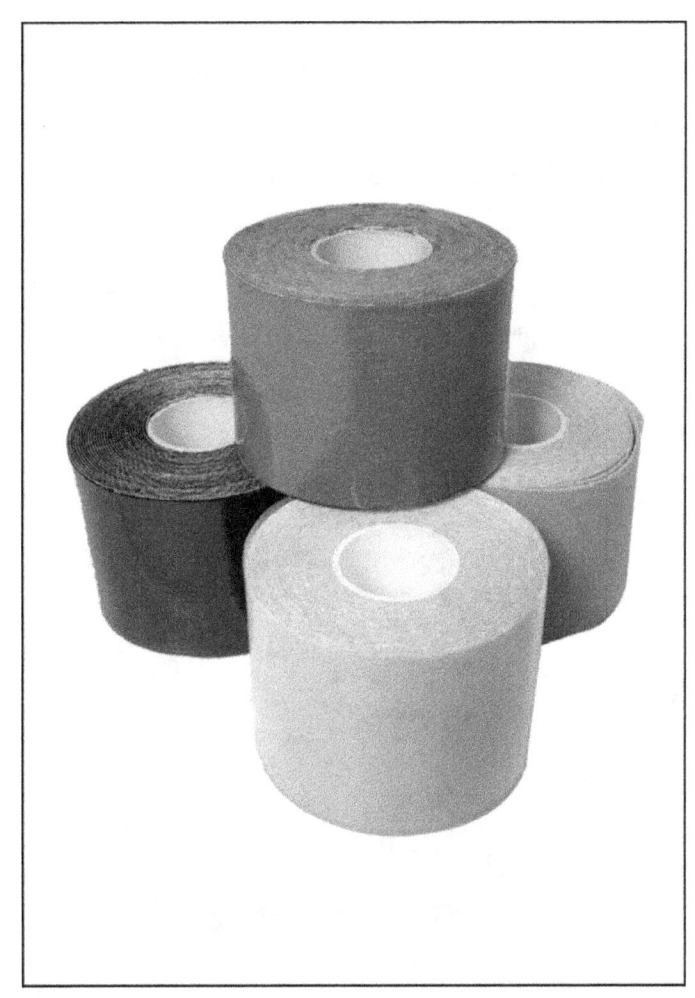

## Kinesiological Taping

Kinesiological taping is a rehabilitative cum protective use of stretchable kinesiological tapes to provide reduction of pain, enhancing performance, preventing injuries, support to the joints, repositioning of structure as well and for fascial and ligamentous correction.[11,33] It facilitates the healing process while providing full range of motion with support to the joint's supportive structures as well as mobilization effects. Kinesiological tapes are widely used in nearly all sports injuries, orthopedic conditions, neurological rehabilitation as well as gynaelogical and pediatric conditions.[70, 76]

The kinesiological tapes are being used in field games, hospitals, clinics and rehabilitation homes. Unlike standard athletic taping, which often involves wrapping a joint for support and compression, kinesiological tape is placed in a variety of patterns depending on the injury. It is pulled into differing degrees of tension to create the desired effect and is typically worn for two to five days, unlike standard tape, which is used mainly during an activity.[45, 52]

Kinesiological taping is best used as an adjunct to physical therapy and exercise. It can unimaginably speed up the rehabilitation process by lessening pain, providing support and correction and also improving tolerance to exercise and movement. The success of Kinesiological taping strongly depends on therapist knowledge and skills[90]. A thorough examination and use of clinical reasoning to find out the structure at fault is integral to determine which taping techniques are indicated. For instance, the clinician must know if the patient needs taping to assist muscle strengthening or to assist muscle relaxation, as the taping will be different. A good physiotherapy rehabilitation protocol goes hand-in-hand with proper taping and evaluation or assessment.

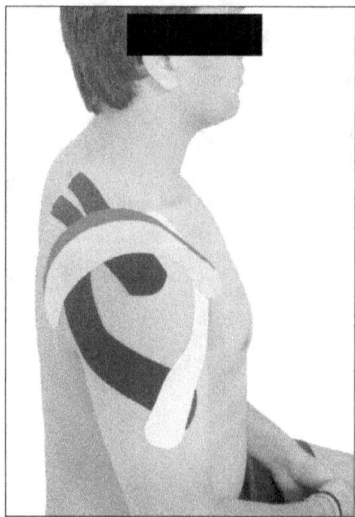

Figure1.1: Kinesiological tapes application for shoulder impingement syndrome.

**Properties of Kinesiological Tapes**

Kinesiological Tapes are made up of cotton, and contains small amount to no latex. The kinesiological tapes are 100% medication free and provide only physical effects not any medical effects so making it a non-side effective therapy. It has a light adhesive made from 100% acrylic, which is almost hypo allergic.

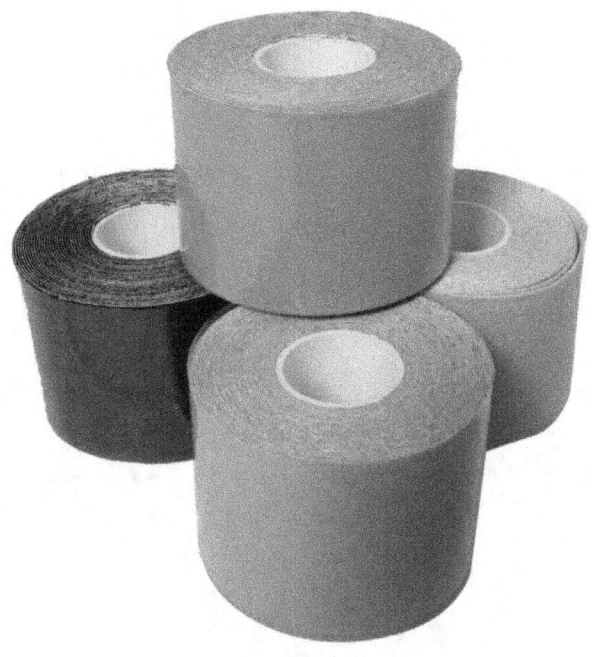

Figure1.2: Kinesiological tapes.

Kinesiological tapes come in different sizes as 5cm X 5m, 2.5cm X 5m, 3.75cm x 5m, 7.5 cm x 5m, but the commonly used tape size is 5cm x 5m which has approximately 8-15 applications depending on the structure and condition to be treated. Kinesiological Tapes are available in various colors ranging from beige, blue, black, pink, red, orange, purple etc. This color difference is only for the psychological factors like light colors are soothing and bright colors are aggressive and boosting. There are no effect on the quality and stretch ability of the tapes of different colors. They all possess the same properties and qualities.

Kinesiological tape stretches to approximately 140%-150% of its original length. That means if we take a strip of 10 cm length, on stretching it can be maximally stretched up to 15 cm in total that is 10 cm original and 50% the total length. This concept has to be understood before starting taping technique, during application we use words like 10% stretch or 100% stretch which literally mean 10% of the available stretch. That means if we say 10% stretch it will corresponds to only 5% of increase in original length. The kinesiological tapes come with 10% pre-stretched length. This pre-stretched length is always kept in mind while removing the backing paper as during application we can use this 10% stretch.

Kinesiological tapes consist of 100% acrylic which is a hypo allergic substance, making it suitable for application to all the individuals. The acrylic glue is masked on the tape in a fixed sine wave pattern. The cotton tape is woven such like that it can only be stretched in a particular longitudinal direction, and not in a transverse direction, this specific acrylic design helps in using the tape to increase or decrease the muscle tone as well as for functional correction. The energy stored in the tape on stretching is only used in one direction, which decreases the wasting of energy. When the tape is stretched it stores the potential energy, now due to its ability to stretch and recoil in longitudinal manner, all the potential energy is used in a specific direction, minimizing the energy loss as well as increasing the efficacy of the tapes.

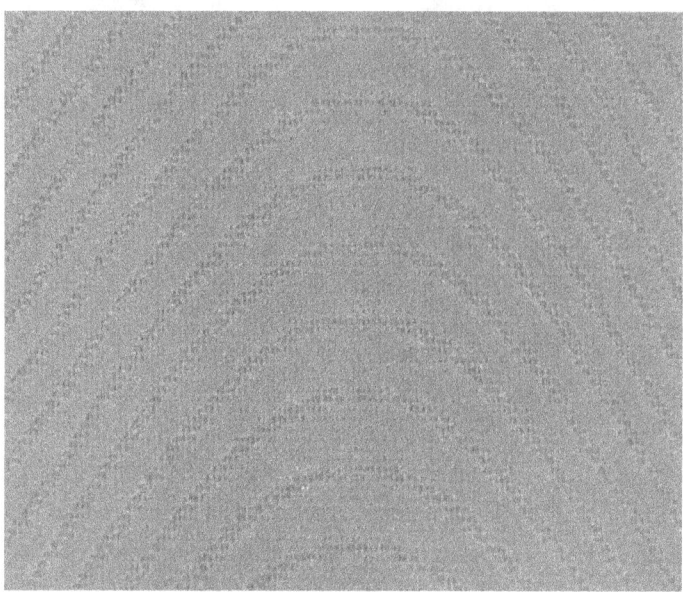

Figure 1.3: Kinesiological tape acrylic glue pattern.

The acrylic adhesive is heat activated. To activate the glue, rub the tape after application so as the therapist feels the warmth; this heat activates the glue and leads to proper adherence of tape onto the skin. It can be easily removed and leaves no sticky residue. Moisture dissipates quickly through the porous material of the tape. Due to its water resistant and hypo allergic properties it can be worn from 2 to 5 days after application.

**Effects of Kinesiological Tape:**

The Kinesiological Taping is a therapeutic taping technique which not only offers the patient and player the support, but also the rehabilitation. By targeting different receptors within the somatosensory system, kinesiological tape alleviates pain and facilitates lymphatic drainage by microscopically lifting the skin. This lifting affect forms convolutions in the skin thus increasing interstitial space and allowing a decrease in inflammation of the affected areas.

Effects of Kinesiological taping:

- Stimulate or inhibit muscle function.
- Enhances proprioception.
- Support joints.
- Fascial correction.
- Pain relief.
- Enhances lymphatic drainage.

**Stimulate or inhibit muscle function:**

Kinesiological tape's elastic properties can be used either to assist muscles during contraction, or inhibit their contraction. When the aim of application of tape is to provide or enhance muscle contraction, the tape base is applied without any stretch to the origin of the muscle, and then the muscle is taken into a stretched position and the tape is applied with no stretch or 10% stretch along the course of muscle. Due to recoil property and sine wave pattern of the glue and a fixed base, the tape will recoils toward the base i.e. its origin, hence facilitating the muscle contraction[11].

When we need to get the inhibition of the muscle activity, we tape the muscle with the base at insertion with no stretch and then keeping the muscle in stretched position, tape is applied throughout the length of muscle till origin, this helps in relieving or inhibiting the muscle activity and is helpful in decreasing the tone and increasing the length of shortened muscles[33,47,76,83].

**Enhances proprioception:**

Kinesiological tapes can be used to create pressure over ligaments and tendons to improve proprioception and dynamic stability. This also has been theorized to stimulate mechanoreceptors; thus improving proprioception. Proprioception means "sense of self". In the limbs, the proprioceptors are sensors that provide information about joint angle, muscle length, and muscle tension, which is integrated to give information about the position of the limb in space. The muscle spindle is one type of proprioceptors that provides information about changes in muscle length. The Golgi tendon organ is another type of proprioceptors that provides information about changes in muscle tension. Thus when the tape is applied it sends the stimulus either by inhibiting or facilitating the muscle action to the brain and helps in enhanced proprioception[61,85].

**Support joints:**

Kinesiological taping is very useful in supporting and protecting the joints while providing complete range of motion. The supporting structure of a joint such as ligament can be taped with ligamentous taping technique so as to provide more stability and support to the ligaments and joint hence preventing injury. The individual ligament can be taped or the group of the ligaments (knee) can also be taped in a circumferential method so as to get joint stability[61].

**Fascial correction:**

Fascia is an intricate web of connective tissue that envelops the entire body underneath the skin, connecting muscles, bones, vessels, organs and more. When fascia becomes dysfunctional or tight, it affects the entire body and can cause altered movement patterns which can lead to injury or further dysfunction. The fascia is divided in three major layers in: the superficial fascia (directly beneath the skin), the deep fascia (surrounding the muscles), and the sub-serous fascia (supporting the internal organs). The fascia surrounds muscles, groups of muscles, blood vessels, and nerves, binding some structures together, while permitting others to slide smoothly over each other. When there is any pathology between the fascia and the structure like muscle, there are formation of adhesion between the fascia and muscle, which will restrict the normal function of the muscle. The elastic properties of the kinesiological tapes can be used as myofascial release as well as it can last the effect, as it has an application time of 2-5 days. While application, the therapist fixes the base and applies a passive stretch or rhythmical correction to fascia and tape the structure with about 80% to 100% stretch. It not only helps in myofascial release but the effects are prolonged[10,21,49,69].

**Pain relief:**

Kinesiological tape is commonly applied to injured or painful muscles while the muscle is in stretched position, when the muscle or tissue is returned to its resting length after tape is applied, wrinkles are created in the taped area because of the elastic property of the tape and the potential energy stored in the tape. These wrinkles are the indication of lifting of the skin. This result in creating a space beneath the skin increasing area for blood and lymph to flow which in result relieves the pain by washing away the waste as well promotes healing. The tape also acts on the mechanoreceptors of the skin causing the relief in pain via the pain gate mechanism[22,26,47].

**Enhancing lymphatic drainage:**

The kinesiological tape application for lymphatic drainage is a fan shaped tape specially designed to reduce swelling, bruising and pain. Its unique "fan shaped" design allows it to be positioned directly over the lymphatic channels responsible for removing excess fluids from the body. The tape exerts a lifting action on the skin, allowing fluid to drain more effectively. As the swelling recedes, this reduces irritation to pain receptors under the skin, leading to relief of pain in severely swollen areas[30].

**Application:**

Kinesiological taping is used as therapeutic cum rehabilitative modality in physiotherapy protocols. Prior to application of any of the therapeutic modality the pre requisite is proper evaluation of the patient or the subject. Merely naming a disease is not the evaluation, the use of clinical reasoning in evaluating helps to determine the structure at fault, which is the basic for accepting the type of tape pattern used. In the conventional taping method via stretchable tape using its complete stretch, the main aim was to limit the range of motion, function of joint or for protection from injury or re-injury. But using the concept of kinesiological taping is entirely different as it enhances or inhibits the muscle, support a structure and it allows protection in full range of motion.

**Clinical Comparisons**

|  | Conventional taping | Kinesiological Taping |
|---|---|---|
| Muscle weakness | Holds | Improves via elastic input |
| Pain | No effect on nociceptors | Stimulates analgesics effects in the skin |
| Muscle spasm | Unloads/holds | Relieves |
| Odema | May restrict fluid flow | Assists fluid flow |
| Range of motion | Limits motion | Assists motion |
| Joint mechanics | Immobilizes | Gives input to joint receptors |
| Length of wear | 1-2 days | Several days |

**Preparation of patient**

The skin should be washed and properly dried. The skin should be free of oils and lotions. Oil or dirt will limit the acrylic adhesive's ability to adhere to the skin, and also limit both effectiveness and duration of application. For some subjects body hair limit adhesion. If the body hair limits adhesion then the therapist needs to shave the area to be treated. In the area where there is moisture and more perspiration, a water resistant solution, or gel is pre applied. This will limit the moisture and help in proper adhesion of the tape.

**Position of the patient**

The patient should be comfortably positioned in such a way that the part to be taped is freely movable. For example: for the application of tape on a deltoid, patient must be seated on a stool, or a couch in a high sitting position so as he/she can perform movement in full range. Similarly is case of ankle, patient can be allowed to lie on the couch with foot and ankle out of the couch and even the long sitting position can be used.

**Position of the therapist**

The position of the therapist depends on the part to be treated and the course of muscle on which tape to be applied. The therapist should adopt such a position from where he can cover the course of muscle, ligament or the structure to be taped. For example: for tape application to the trapezius upper fibers, the therapist can stand in front or back of the patient, similarly in case of application of tape to sciatic nerve course therapist usually stand in front of patient while the patient is in side lying position and therapist holds the extremity.

**Kinesiological tape strips**

Types of strips commonly used in kinesiological taping

- I strip
- Y strip
- X strip
- I Strip with hole
- X strip with hole
- Fan shaped

"I" shaped strips are commonly used strip during kinesiological taping, "I" strip is the required length of the tape, with its end rounded off. "I" strips are used for muscle application, ligament techniques and space correction techniques.

"Y" Strip is a modified "I" strip which has a single base but is cut into two vertical strips from either end. The length of vertical cut depends on the length of muscle belly, for e.g. taping for extensor pollicis longus , the muscle has a short belly and a long tendons end, the "I" strip is cut into the "Y" till the length of muscle belly and the tendinous part is taped with base or single strip. "Y" strips are used for muscle as well as for fascial correction and mechanical correction techniques.

"X" strips are modified "Y" strip, which has a single centre and bifurcated from the both ends. "X" strips also called as "double "Y" shaped". It is used in the areas where there is two joint muscle application technique and the level of stretch differs with the courses of the muscles.

"I" and "X" strips with hole at center are modification of these strip where there is a triangular hole in the middle of the strips, these are used in taping of area with bony prominence so as there is no restriction of the movement, for example, as in taping for olecronon bursitis, "I" strip and "X" are used at posterior aspect of elbow, so as to facilitate the extension, we cut a hole in center so as there is no restriction to olecronon movement.

Fan shaped strips have a single base on one side, the other side its spilled or cut into 4 or 6 strips making it look like a hand fan, or multiple "Y" strips. These are used specifically for lymphatic application. It helps in activation of lymphatic ducts, improving circulation by creating space beneath the skin.

Pictures of tapes:

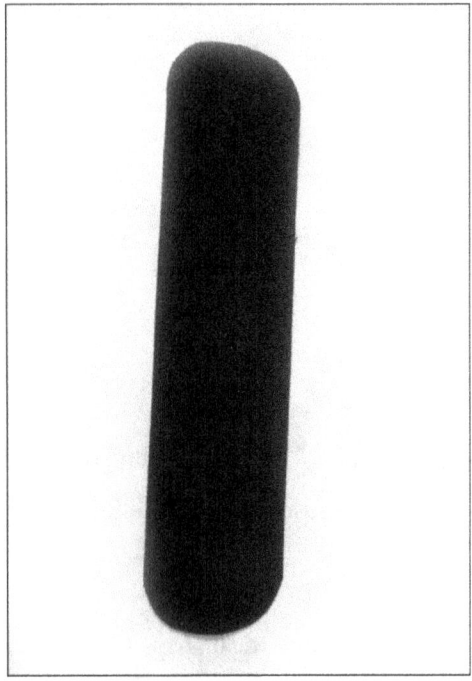

Figure 1.4: "I" strip.

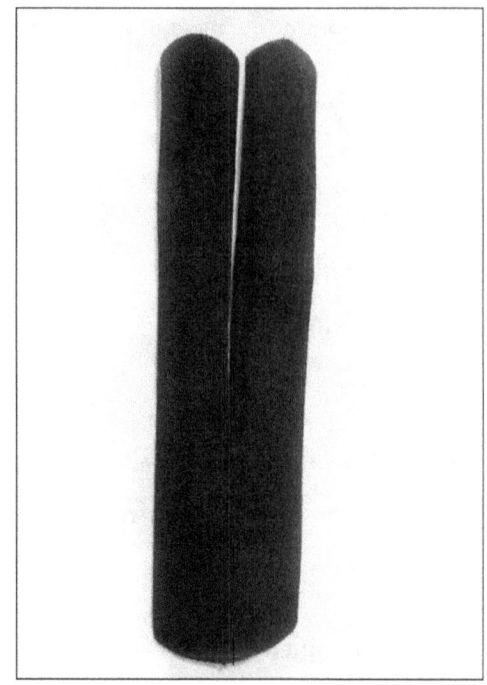

Figure 1.5: "Y" strip.

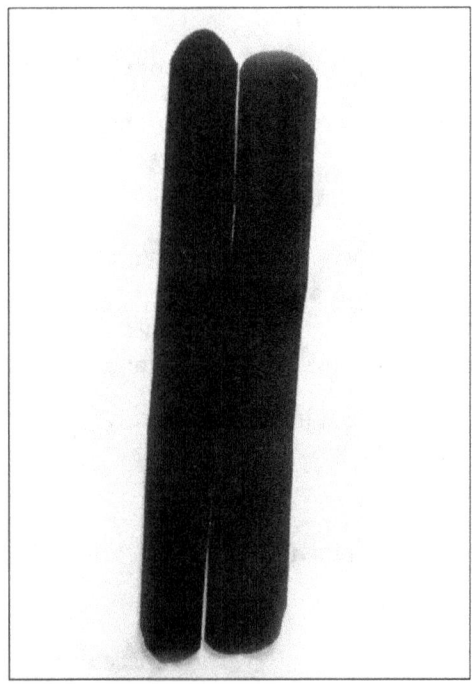

Figure 1.6: "X" strip.

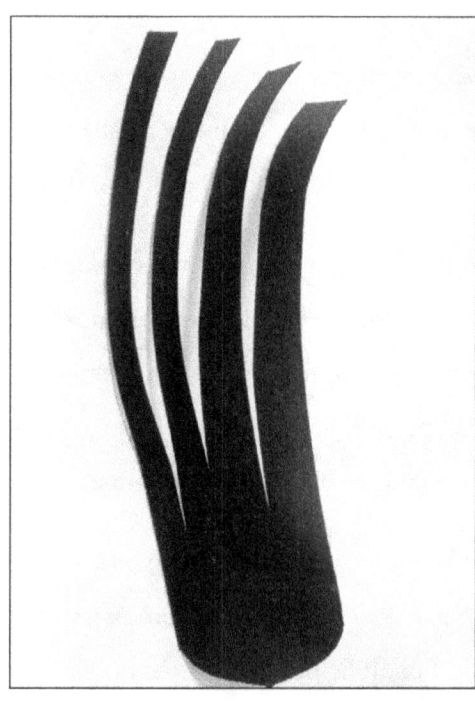

Figure 1.7: "FAN" strip.

**Removal of Backing Paper:**

The removal of tape from the backing paper is one of the most important parts for proper application of the tape. The therapist must take every possible precaution to avoid touching the adhesive side of the tape.

There are two ways to remove the backing paper which depends on the type of application being used:

1.  Application of base: The therapist must hold the tape strip vertically and by the use of the index finger just strip of the edge of backing paper, so as just a corner is exposed, now the tape is removed so that the part that is the base is exposed from the paper, the backing paper is folded back prior to application of base, and then the base is fixed on the part to be treated. This removal technique is used in muscle application.

2.  Application of center: This technique is mainly used in ligament correction, or in space taping procedures where we need to apply the middle part first then the base. The therapist holds the strip horizontally with both hands, tearing the center of tape with paper, this result in tearing the backing paper not the tape, the backing paper is folded back and the tape is applied with even stretch to the part.

**Pictures of removing of backing paper:**

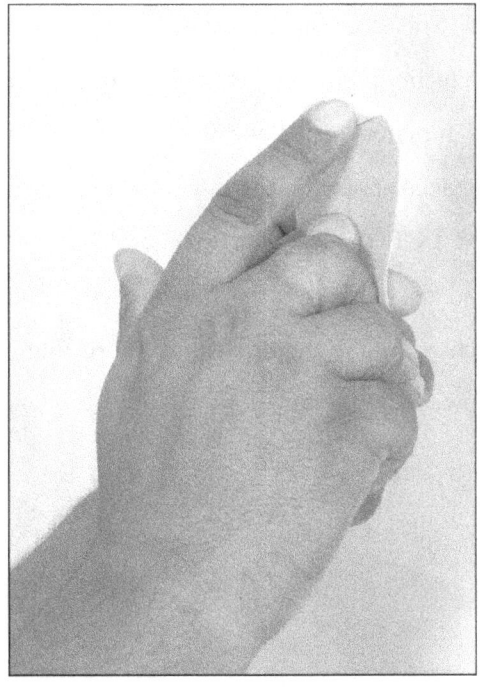

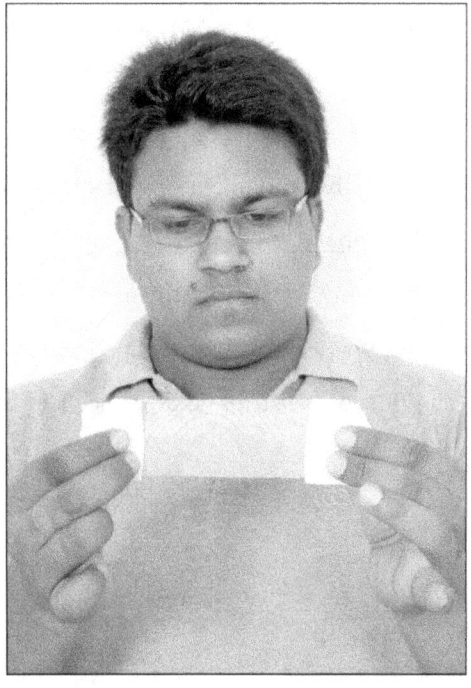

Figure 1.8: Removal of backing paper.        Figure 1.9: Tearing of backing paper from center.

**Four Taping Techniques 4TT's:**

- Muscle Taping Technique (MTT).
- Ligament Taping Technique (LTT).
- Fascia Correction Taping Technique (FCTT).
- Lymphatic Corrective Taping Technique (LCTT).

Taping techniques has been classified into four basic groups depending on the structures and outcome for which taping is to be done.

1. <u>Muscle Taping Technique (MTT)</u>: These taping techniques as understood by name, and are used to tape the muscular structures. In muscle taping, two techniques are used depending on the desired outcome: tonus up and tonus down technique.

2. <u>Ligament Taping Technique (LTT)</u>: Ligament taping is used to reinforce the ligamentous structure, with all the stretch maintained at center of tape. Ligament technique is also used as tendon technique and space technique.

   <u>Space Taping Techniques (STT)</u>: This technique is used in the acute injury conditions, painful areas and for trigger points. The principle of STT is to use the recoil property of the tape to create space beneath the skin so as to promote flow of fluids and reducing pain by decreasing pressure as well.

3. <u>Fascia Correction Taping Technique (FCTT)</u>: This technique works on the biomechanical alignment of the structures like fascia and bones. This technique is used to correct a functional abnormality. FCTT is used as a corrective technique or a repositioning technique where aim is to realign or correct a biomechanical function of a bone like patella or for corrective alignment of vertebrae or for correction of fascial abnormality.

4. <u>Lymphatic Correction Taping Technique (LCTT)</u>: The LCTT is used to correct and increase the flow of lymph towards the lymphatic ducts so as to reduce the lymphodema and lymphstasis. The fan shaped strips are applied which stimulate the ducts and the recoiling effect of the strips create space and enhance lymph flow.

# CHAPTER 2

# MUSCLE TAPING TECHNIQUES

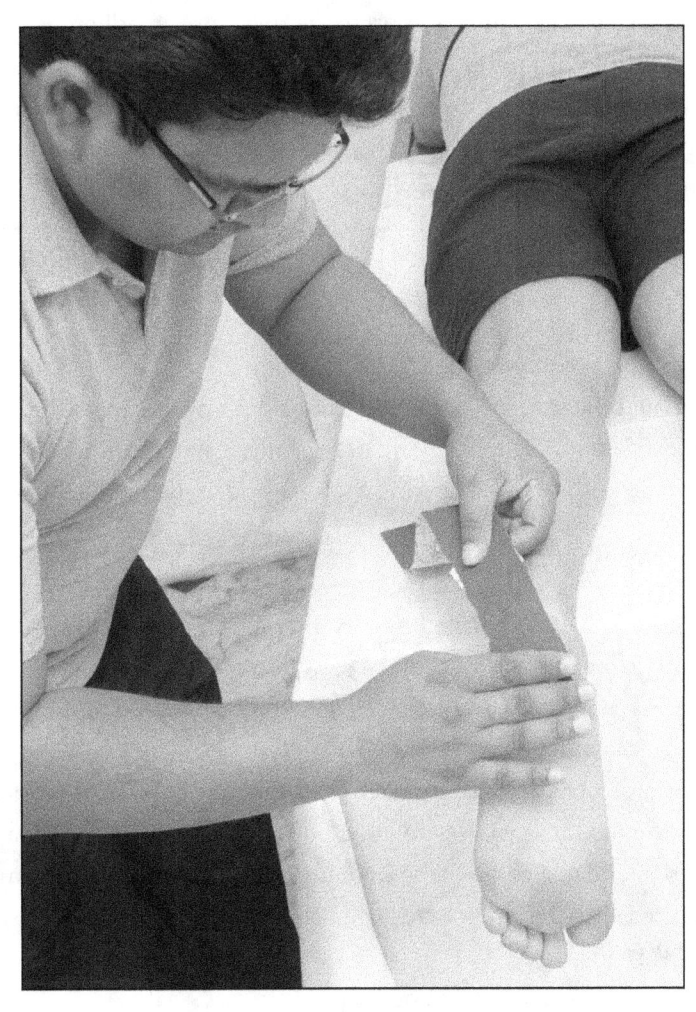

# Muscle Taping Technique

Muscle Taping Techniques (MTT)

The muscle taping techniques are based on the properties of the skeletal muscles i.e. the tone of the muscle. MTT can be used for decreasing or increasing the tone of the muscle, or more precisely to increase or decrease the length of the muscle.[83,76].

These are being classified as:

    a. Tonus up techniques.
    b. Tonus down techniques.

**Tonus up Taping Technique:**

Generally the "I" and "Y" strips are used for tonus up taping technique. Primary step of every taping technique is to measure the tape. The tape is measured from origin to insertion of the muscle with muscle in stretched position, the measured tapes are cut and the ends are rounded off from both the sides. Rounding off the edges is of utmost important as this helps in adherence of tape to the skin for long time. The basic principle of taping for increasing the tone is to apply the tape from origin of muscle to its insertion. The base of the tape is applied just 1-2 cm proximal to the origin of muscle, the base is applied without stretch, the muscle is then taken into the stretched position while therapist applies the tape to the course of the muscle with paper off, tension or 10% stretch on the tails. Just before the application of end of the tape, the subject is again asked to take the muscle in neutral position, and then the end of the tape is applied without stretch.[11,83]

**Action of tape:**

As the base is on origin and the stretch is applied from origin towards insertion, the sine wave pattern of the tape is also stretched, now due to recoiling of the tape, it will recoil towards the base, displacing the skin towards the origin and hence facilitating the tone and assisting the muscular contraction.[11]

General steps for tonus up techniques:

- Evaluation: This is the prerequisite of every therapy, the subject must be evaluated and the structure at fault is diagnosed followed by selection of taping technique.
- Part of the subject should be completely clean from dirt and oil and in case of excessive body hair, it should be shaved off.
- Measuring the tape: The subject is asked to keep the muscle in stretched position or the therapist will take the muscle into stretched position and the length of tape is measured from origin to insertion and just cut the tape 2 cm more from the measured length.
- Select the required strip design, for large muscle belly the "Y" strips is used and in flat muscle generally the "I" strip is used.
- The corners of the tapes are rounded off.
- Application of base: Apply the base with no stretch just 2 cm proximal the origin while the subject is in neutral position or the resting position.

- Application of the tail: While subject is in stretch muscle position, the base is stabilized with one hand while the therapist applies the rest of the tape with paper off or 10% stretch.
- At the end of application rub the tape until the warmth is felt, this is necessary to activate the glue.

**Tonus down Taping Technique:**

Generally the "I" and "Y" strips are used for tonus down taping technique. Primary step of every taping technique is to measure the tape. The tape is measured from insertion to origin of the muscle with muscle in stretched position, the measured tapes are cut and the ends are rounded off from both the sides. Rounding off the edges is of utmost important as it helps in adherence of tape to the skin for long time. The basic principle of taping for decreasing the tone is to tape the muscle from insertion to the origin. The base of the tape is applied just 1-2 cm distal to the insertion of muscle, the base is applied without stretch, the muscle is then taken into the stretched position while therapist apply the tape to the course of the muscle with paper off tension or 10% stretch on the tails. Just before the application of end of the tape, the subject is again asked to take the muscle in neutral position, and then the end of the tape is applied.[83]

**Action of tape:**

As the base is on insertion and the stretch is applied from insertion towards origin, the sine wave pattern of the tape is also stretched, now due to recoiling property of the tape, it will recoil towards the base, displacing the skin towards the insertion and hence inhibiting the tone and muscular contraction[11].

General steps for tonus down techniques:

1. Evaluation: This is the prerequisite of every therapy, the subject must be evaluated and the structure at fault is diagnosed and selection of taping technique is done.
2. Part of the subject should be completely clean from dirt and oil and in case of excessive body hair, it should be shaved off.
3. Measuring the tape: The subject is asked to be in a muscle stretch position or the therapist take the muscle into stretched position and the length of tape is measured from insertion to origin and just cut the tape 2cm more from the measured length.
4. Select the required strip design, for large muscle belly the "Y" strip is used and in flat muscle generally the "I" strip is used.
5. The corners of the tapes are rounded off.
6. Application of base: Apply the base with no stretch just 2 cm distal to the insertion while the subject is in neutral position or the muscle is in resting position.
7. Application of the tail: While subject is in stretch muscle position, the base is stabilized with one hand while the therapist applies the rest of the tape with paper off or 10% stretch.
8. At the end of application rub the tape until the warmth is felt, this is necessary to activate the glue.

## Scalenus

**Technique Used:** Tonus down muscle technique.

**Muscle:** Scalene[67].

**Origin:**

- Anterior tubercles of the transverse processes of vertebrae C3-C6.

**Insertion:**

- Scalene tubercle of the first rib.

**Innervations:** The brachial plexus, C5-C7.

**Function:**

- Elevates the first rib;
- Flexes and laterally bends the neck.

**Subject Position:** Subject sitting in relaxed comfortable position.

**Therapist Position:** Therapist standing behind the subject.

**Strip:** Y strip is used.

**Procedure:**

- Follow the basic steps for muscle taping.
- Measuring the tape: The subject is asked to side flex the neck and the tape is measured from root of neck to the mastoid process (Fig: 2.1).
- Select the required strip design, for large muscle bulk, use "I" strip and in small muscle generally the "Y" strip.
- The corners of the tapes are rounded off.
- Application of base: Apply the base with no stretch just on lateral surface of neck starting from root of neck (Fig: 2.2).
- Application of the tail: When subject's muscle is in stretched position, therapist stabilizes the base with one hand and applies the rest of the tape with paper off or 10% stretch. (Fig: 2.3).
- At the end of application rub the tape until the warmth is felt, this is necessary to activate the glue.

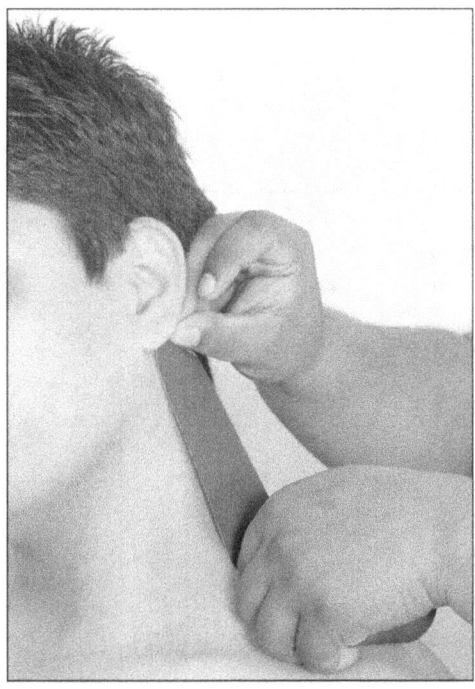

Figure 2.1: Measuring the tape.

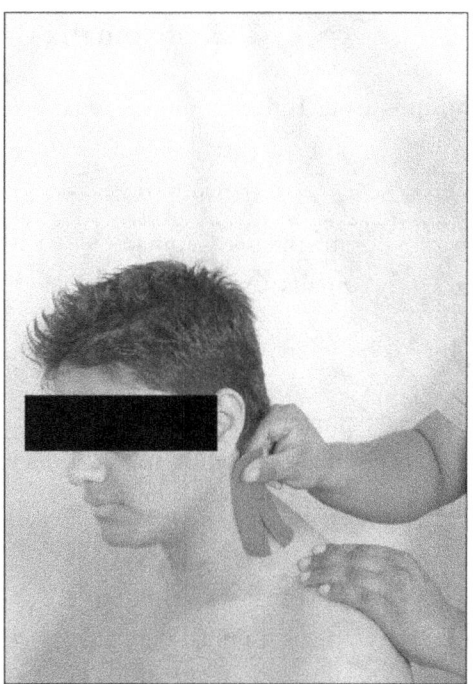

Figure 2.2: Application of base.

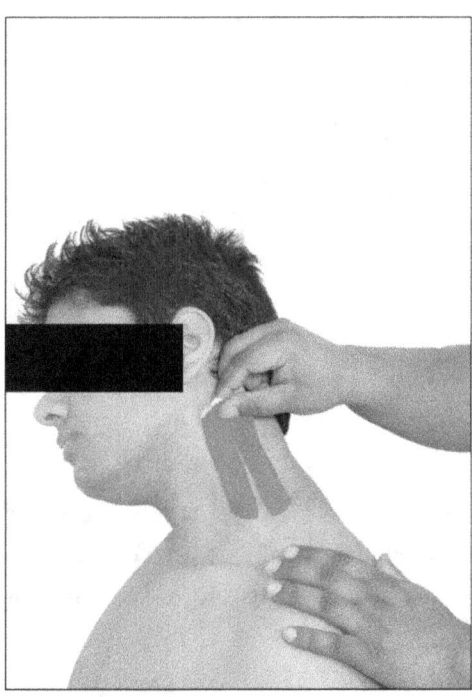

Figure 2.3: Application of tail.

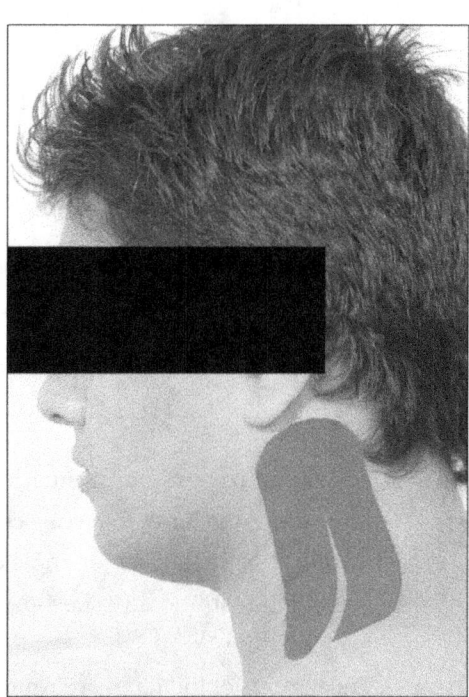

Figure 2.4: Final application.

## Semispinalis Capitis And Spinalis Capitis

**Technique used**: Tonus up muscle technique.

**Muscle**:

- Semispinalis Capitis.[42]
- Spinalis Capitis [42].

**Origin:**

- Semispinalis Capitis - Transverse processes of C7-T12,
- Spinalis Capitis - Spinous processes at inferior vertebral levels.

**Insertion:**

- Semispinalis Capitis: back of skull between nuchal lines,[82]
- Spinalis Capitis - Spinous processes at superior vertebral levels and base of the skull.

**Function:**

- Semispinalis Capitis - Extends the trunk and laterally bends the trunk, rotates the trunk to the opposite side.
- Spinalis Capitis- Extends and laterally bends trunk and neck. ,[82]

**Innervation:**

- Semispinalis Capitis- Dorsal primary rami of spinal nerves C1-T12.
- Spinalis Capitis- Dorsal primary rami of spinal nerves C2-L3,[82]

**Subject's position**: Subject is in sitting position.

**Therapist position:** Therapist is standing at the back of the subject.

**Strip:** Y shaped tape is used.

**Procedure:**

- Follow the basic steps for muscle taping.
- Measuring the tape: The subject is asked to forward flex the neck; the tape is measured from T12 or T8 (at inferior angle of scapula) to just below the hair line at back of the neck.
- Select the required strip design, for large muscle bulk, use "I" strip and in small muscle generally the "Y" strip.
- The corners of the tapes are rounded off.
- Application of base: Apply the base with no stretch just distal to the T 8 vertebrae (Fig: 2.5).
- Application of the tail: When subject's muscle is in stretched position, therapist stabilizes the base with one hand and applies the rest of the tape with paper off or 10% stretch (Fig: 2.6).

- At the end of application rub the tape until the warmth is felt, this is necessary to activate the glue (Fig: 2.7).

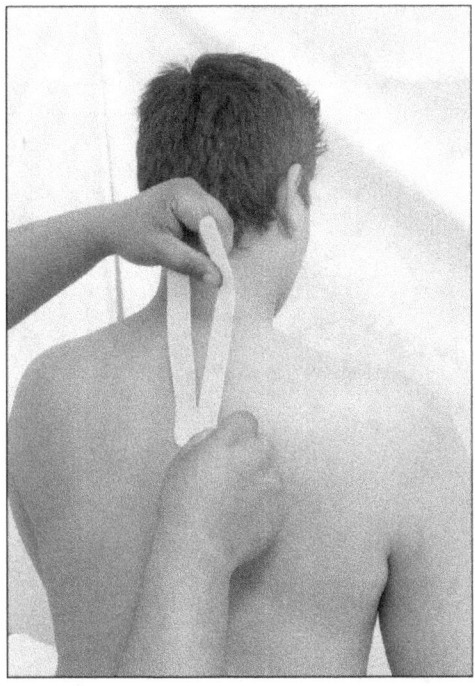

Figure 2.5: Application of base.

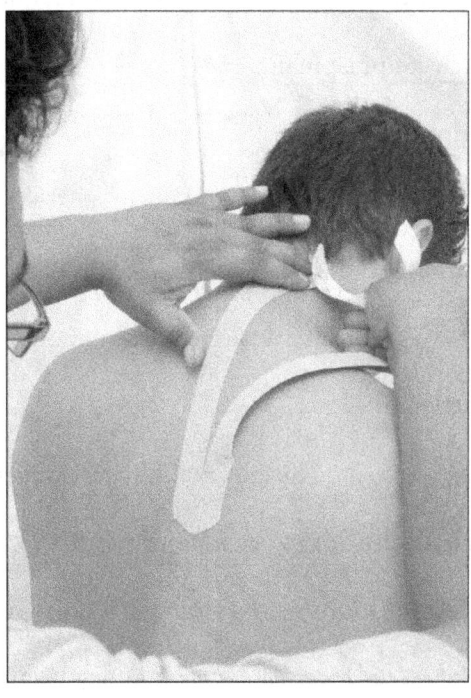

Figure 2.6: Application of tail.

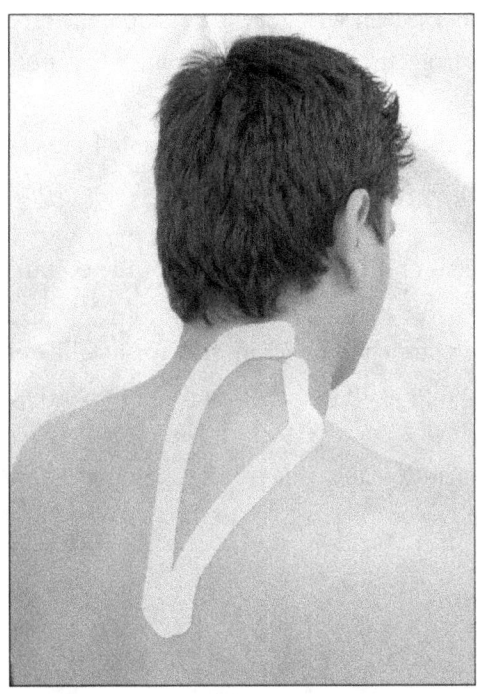

Figure 2.7: Final application.

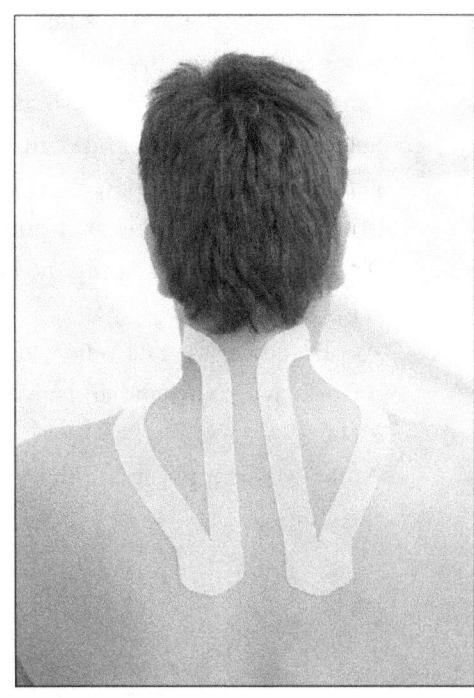

Figure 2.8: Bilateral application.

# Supraspinatus

**Technique Used**: Tonus up muscle technique.

**Muscle**: Supraspinatus[64],[86,92].

**Origin**:

- Supraspinatous Fossa.

**Insertion**:

- Greater tubercle of the humerus[77].

**Function**:

- Abducts the arm (initiates abduction).

**Innervations:** Suprascapular nerve (C5, C6).

**Subject Position**: Subject sitting in relaxed comfortable position.

**Therapist Position**: Therapist standing behind the subject.

**Strip:** Y strip is used.

**Procedure:**

- Follow the basic steps for muscle.
- Measuring the tape: The subject is asked to adduct the arm with forward flexion, the tape is measured from the medial border of scapula from the point where spine of scapula starts to the greater tubercle of humerus (Fig: 2.9).
- Select the required strip design, for large muscle bulk, use "I" strip and in small muscle generally the "Y" strip.
- The corners of the tapes are rounded off.
- Application of base: Apply the base with no stretch on the medial border of the scapula (Fig: 2.10).
- Application of the tail: When subject's muscle is in stretched position, therapist stabilizes the base with one hand and applies the rest of the tape with paper off or 10% stretch (Fig: 2.11).
- At the end of application rub the tape until the warmth is felt, this is necessary to activate the glue.

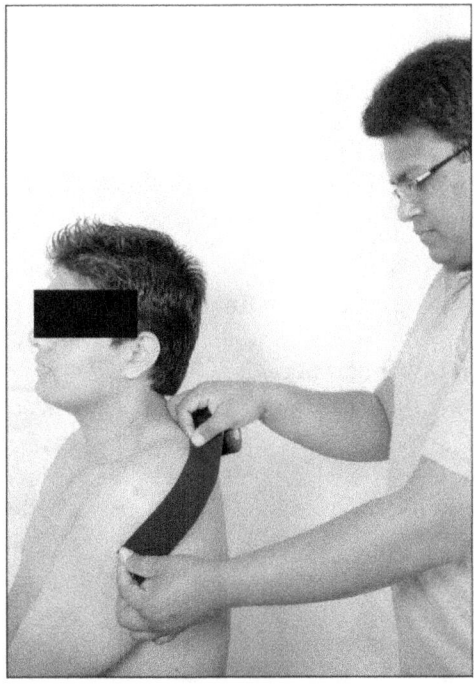

Figure 2.9: Measuring the tape.

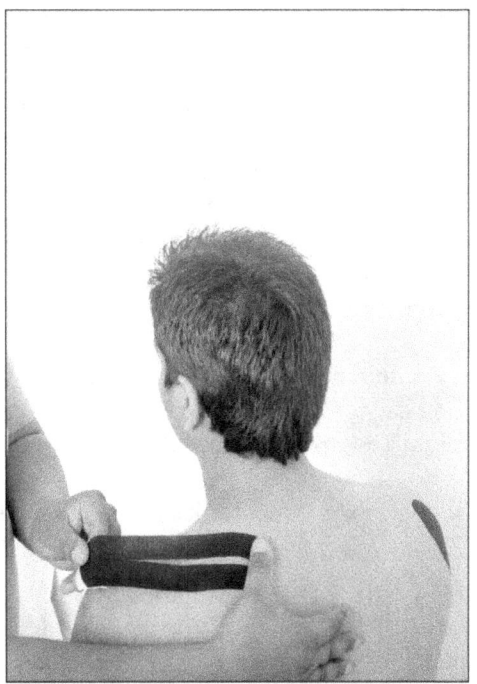

Figure 2.10: Application of base.

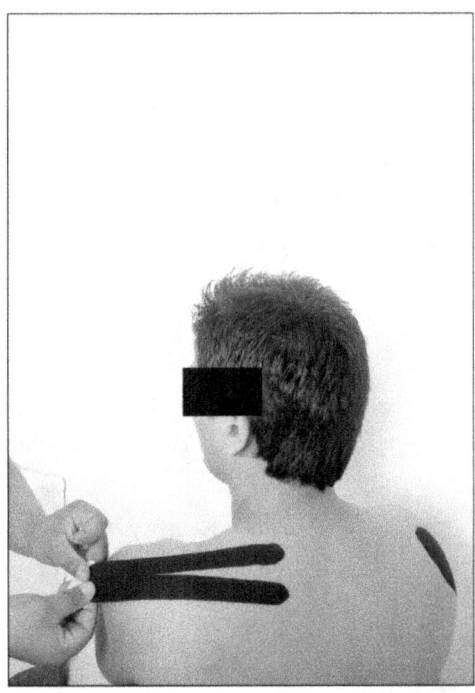

Figure 2.11: Application of tail.

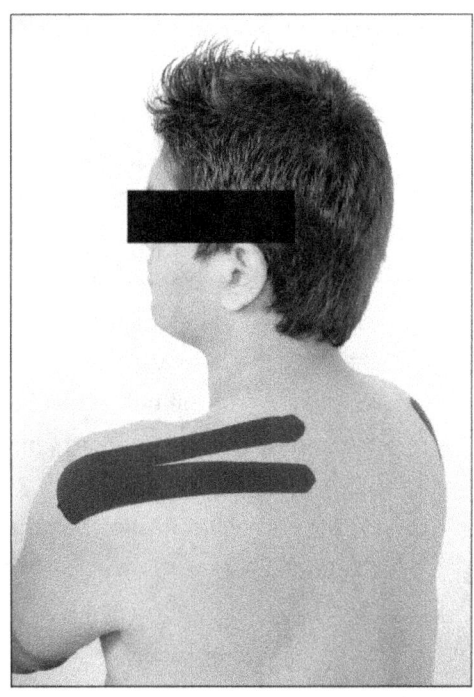

Figure 2.12: Final application.

# Infraspinatus

**Technique used**: Tonus up muscle technique.

**Muscle**: Infraspinatus[64,77,86,92].

**Origin**: The muscle arises from the medial two-thirds of the infraspinatous fossa.

**Insertion**: It insertes into the middle impression on the greater tubercle of the humerus.

**Innervation**: The infraspinatus muscle is innervated by the suprascapular nerve.

**Function:** The primary function of the infraspinatus is:

- Extension, horizontal (transverse) extension and lateral rotation of humerus at the shoulder joint;
- It abducts the inferior angle of the scapula.

**Subject position**: Subject sitting in relaxed comfortable position.

**Therapist position**: Therapist standing behind the subject.

**Strip:** Y-strip is used.

**Procedure:**

- Follow the basic steps for muscle taping.
- Measuring the tape:  The subject is asked to do flexion and internal rotation of the shoulder so as to put the muscle in a stretched position, the tape is measured from medial border of scapula to greater tubercle of the humerus (Fig: 2.13).
- Select the required strip design, for large muscle bulk, use two "I" strip and in small muscle generally the "Y" strip.
- The corners of the tapes are rounded off.
- Application of base: Apply the base with no stretch just 2cm proximal to the origin while the subject is in neutral position or the resting position (Fig: 2.14).
- Application of the tail: When subject's muscle is in stretched position, therapist stablises the base with one hand and applies the rest of the tape with paper off or 10% stretch (Fig: 2.15).
- At the end of application rub the tape until the warmth is felt, this is necessary to activate the glue.

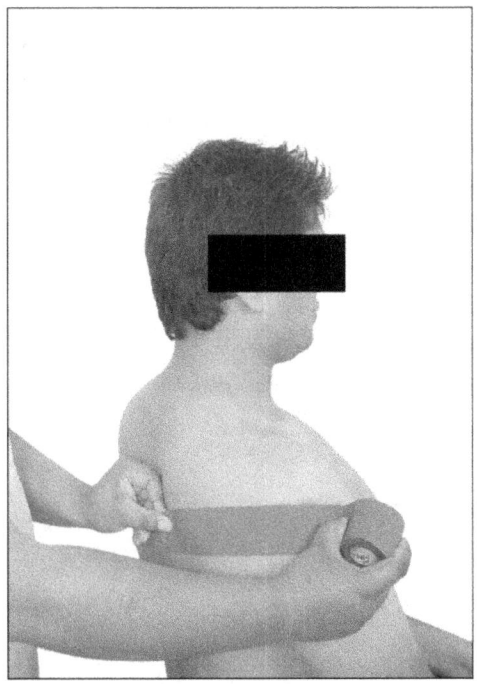

Figure 2.13: Measuring the tape.

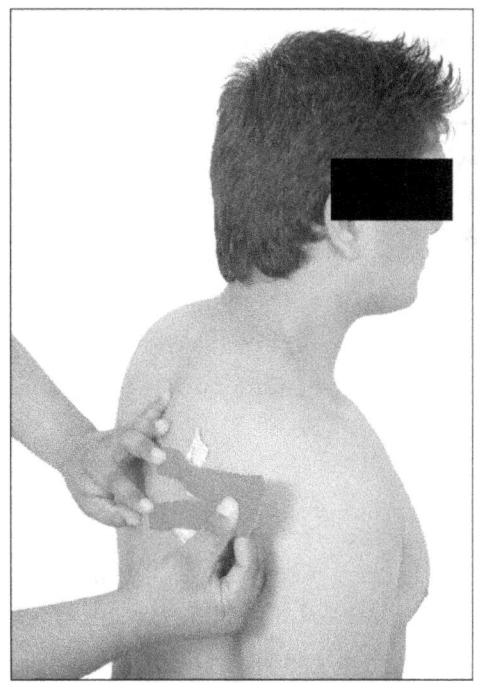

Figure 2.14: Application of base.

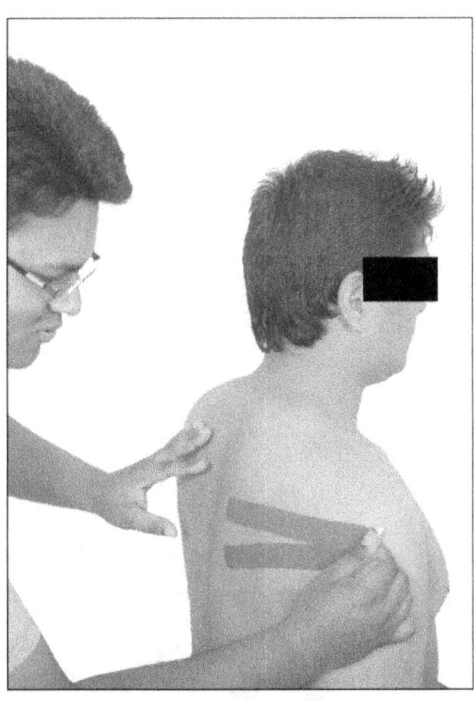

Figure 2.15: Application of tail.

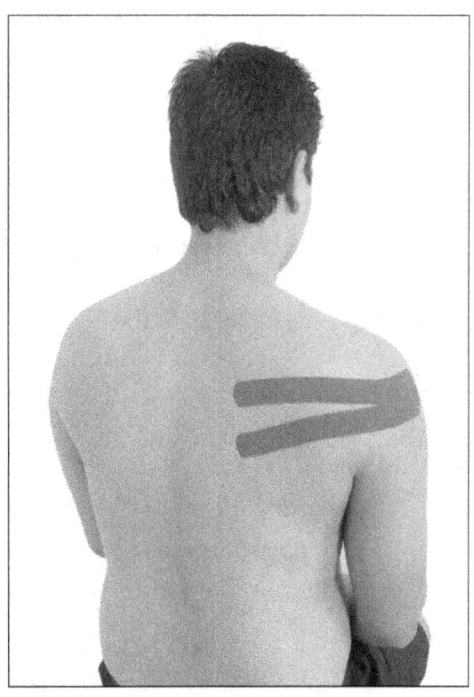

Figure 2.16: Final Application.

## Upper Trapezius & Lower Trapezius

**Technique used:** Upper trapezius muscle tonus down technique and tonus up muscle technique for lower fibers.

**Muscle:** Trapezius[64,77].

**Origin:**

- External occipital protuberance;
- Along the medial sides of the superior nuchal line;
- Ligamentum nuchae (surrounding the cervical spinous processes) spinous processes of C1-T12.

**Insertion:**

- Posterior, lateral 1/3 of clavicle;
- Medial side of the acromion;
- Superior spine of scapula.

**Innervation:** Spinal Accessory (XI) Ventral ramii of C3 & C4.

**Function:**

- Elevates scapula;
- Upward rotation of the scapula (upper fibers);
- Downward rotation of the scapula (lower fibers);
- Retracts scapula.

**Subject position:** Subject sitting in relaxed comfortable position.

**Therapist position:** Therapist standing at the affected side of the subject.

**Strip:** "I" strip is used, for both the fibers.

**Procedure:**

- Follow the basic steps for muscle taping.
- Measuring the tape :
  - Upper trapezius fibers (tonus down technique): The subjects is asked to do side neck flexion, the strip is measured from lower hair line to 2 cm distal to the acromion process (Fig: 2.17).
  - For lower fibers: The subject is asked to do protraction, the strip is measured from medial border of scapula to 2 cm lateral to T12 vertebrae(Fig: 2.21).
- Select the required strip design, for large muscle bulk, use two "I" strip and in small muscle generally the "Y" strip.
- The corners of the tapes are rounded off.
- Application of base:

- For upper fibers: Apply the base with no stretch just 2 cm lateral to the acromion process while the subject is in neutral position or the resting position (Fig: 2.18).
- For lower fibers: Apply the base with no stretch just 2 cm lateral to the T12 vertebrae while the subject is in neutral position or the resting position (Fig: 2.22).

- Application of the tail: When subject's muscle is in stretched position, therapist stabilizes the base with one hand and applies the rest of the tape with paper off or 10% stretch. The stretch position of both fibers will differ (Fig: 2.19, Fig: 2.23).
- At the end of application rub the tape until the warmth is felt, this is necessary to activate the glue.

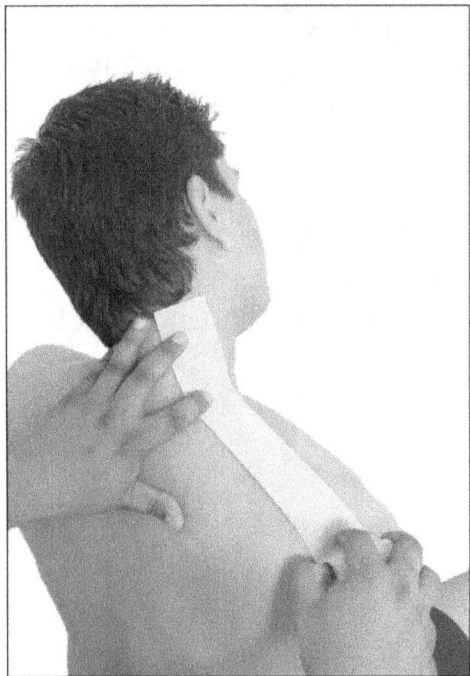

Figure 2.17: Measuring the tape.

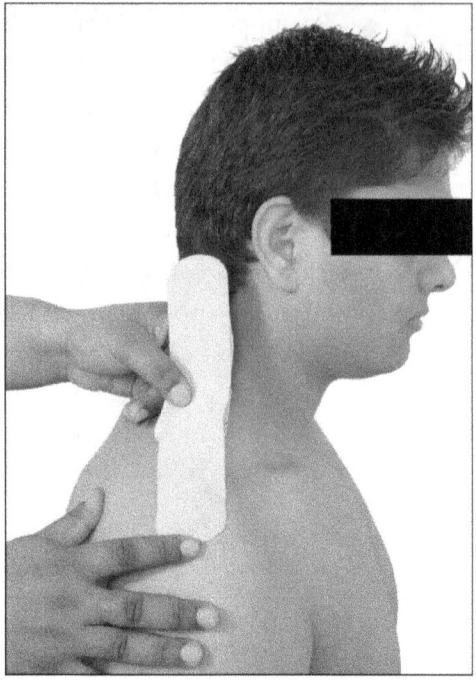

Figure 2.18: Application of base.

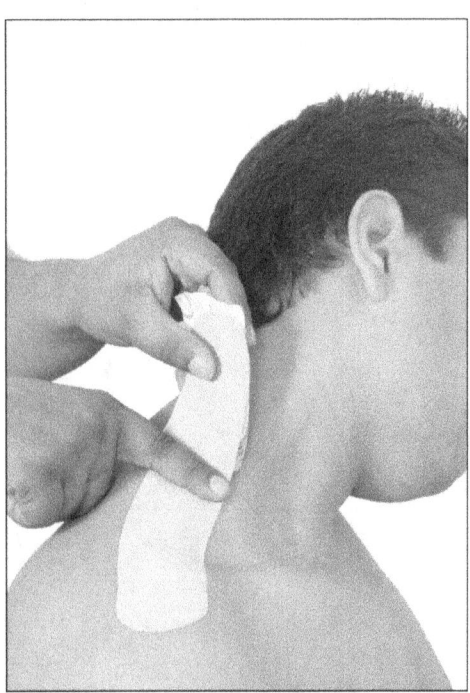

Figure 2.19: Application of tail.

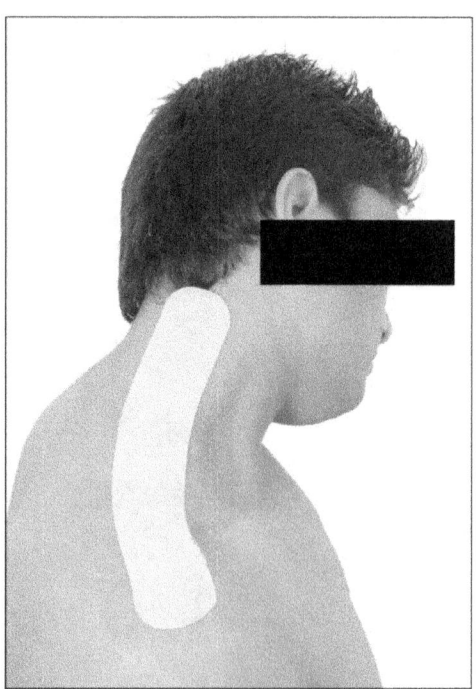

Figure 2.20: Final application.

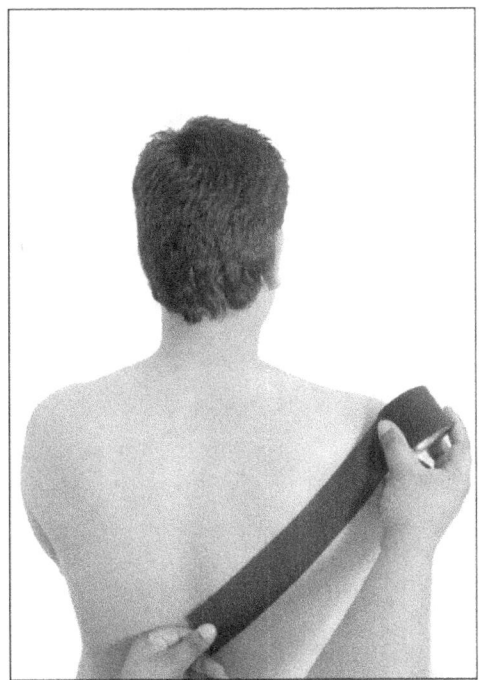

Figure 2.21: Measuring the tape.

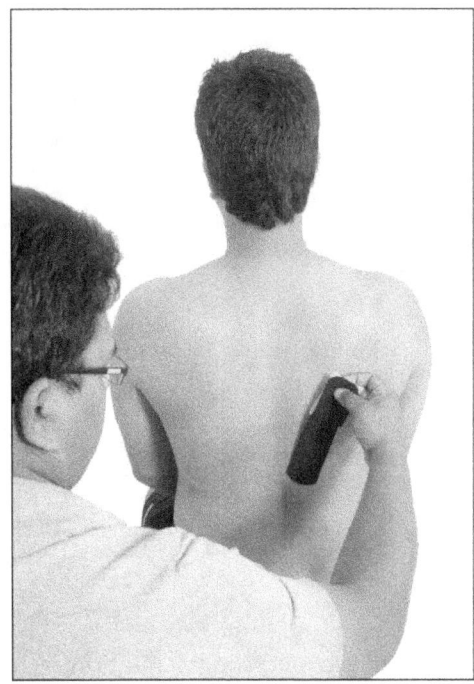

Figure 2.22: Application of base.

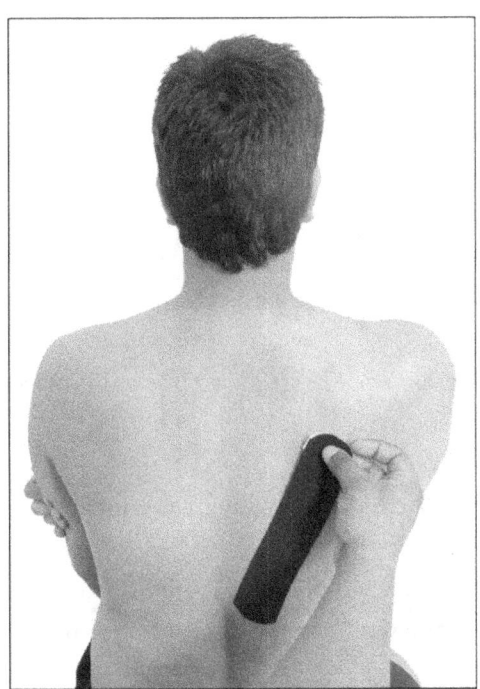

Figure 2.23: Application of tail.

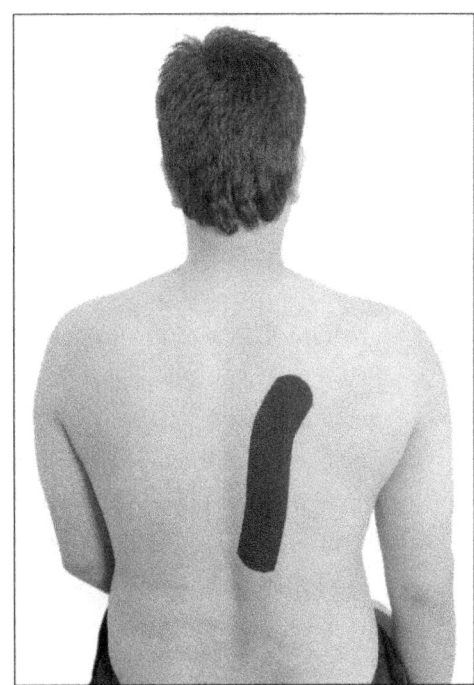

Figure 2.24: Final application.

# Pectoralis Major

**Technique Used**: Muscle tonus down Technique.

**Muscle**: Pectoralis major[48].

**Origin**:

- Medial 1/2 of the clavicle,
- Manubrium & body of sternum,
- Costal cartilages of ribs 2-6.

**Insertion**:

- Crest of the greater tubercle of the humerus.

**Function**:

- Flexes and adducts the arm,
- Medially rotates the arm.

**Innervations**: Medial and Lateral Pectoral Nerves (C5-T1).

**Subject Position**: Subject sitting in relaxed comfortable position.

**Therapist Position**: Therapist standing behind the subject.

**Strip:** Y strip is used.

**Procedure:**

- Follow the basic steps for muscle taping.
- Measuring the tape: The subject is asked to abduct the arm to 90 degrees with lateral rotation of the shoulder, the tape is measured from the 6th rib costal cartilage to the greater tubercle of the humerus (Fig: 2.25).
- Select the required strip design, for large muscle bulk, use "I" strip and in small muscle generally the "Y" strip.
- The corners of the tapes are rounded off.
- Application of base: Apply the base with no stretch 2 cm distal to the greater tubercle of the humerus (Fig: 2.26).
- Application of the tail: When subject's muscle is in stretched position, therapist stabilizes the base with one hand and applies the rest of the tape with paper off or 10% stretch (Fig: 2.27).
- At the end of application rub the tape until the warmth is felt, this is necessary to activate the glue.

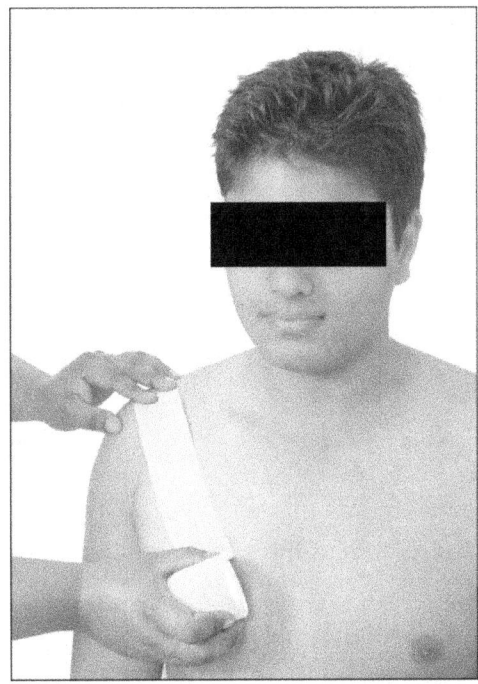

Figure 2.25: Measuring the tape.

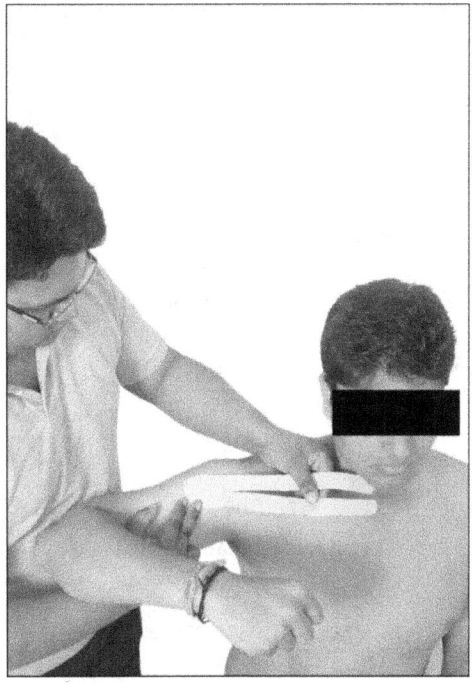

Figure 2.26: Application of base.

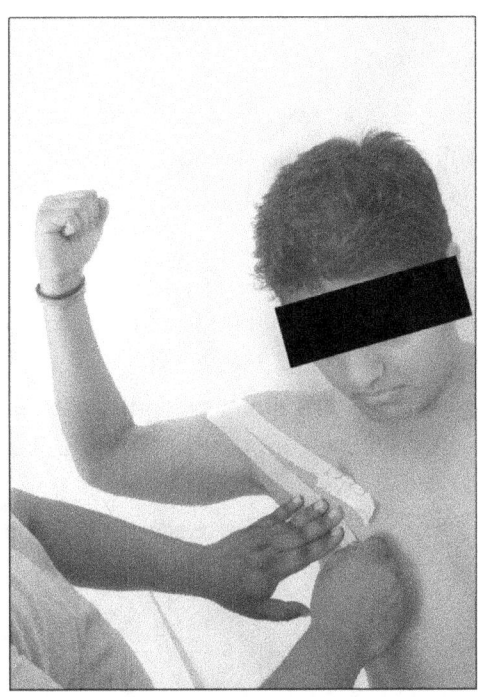

Figure 2.27: Application of tail.

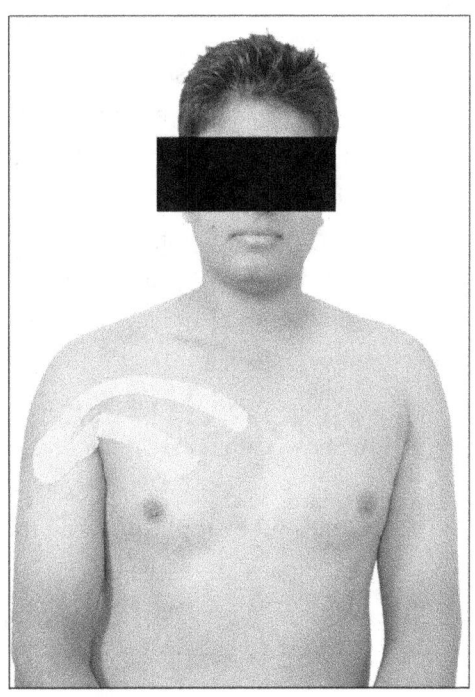

Figure 2.28: Final application.

# Rhomboidus Major

**Technique used**: Tonus up muscle technique.

**Muscle**: Rhomboids major[21,22].

**Origin**: The rhomboid major arises from the spinous processes of the thoracic vertebrae T2 to T5.

**Insertion**: Medial border of the scapula inferior to the spine of the scapula.

**Innervation**: Dorsal scapular nerve.

**Function**: The rhomboids act

- To retract the scapula, pulling it towards the vertebral column ,
- Collectively act with the levator scapulae muscles to elevate the medial border of the scapula,
- To downward rotate the scapula with respect to the glenohumeral joint.

**Subject position**: Subject sitting in relaxed comfortable position.

**Therapist position**: Therapist standing behind the subject.

**Strip:** Y-strip is used.

**Procedure:**

- Follow the basic steps for muscle taping.
- Measuring the tape: The subject is asked to protract the shoulders; the tape is measured 2 cm lateral to the centre of thoracic spine to the medial border of the scapula (Fig: 2.29).
- Select the required strip design, for large muscle bulk, use two "I" strip and in small muscle generally the "Y" strip.
- The corners of the tapes are rounded off.
- Application of base: Apply the base with no stretch just 2 cm lateral to the origin from spine while the subject is in neutral position or the resting position(Fig: 2.30).
- Application of the tail: When subject's muscle is in stretched position, therapist stablises the base with one hand and applies the rest of the tape with paper off or 10% stretch (Fig: 2.31).
- At the end of application rub the tape until the warmth is felt, this is necessary to activate the glue.

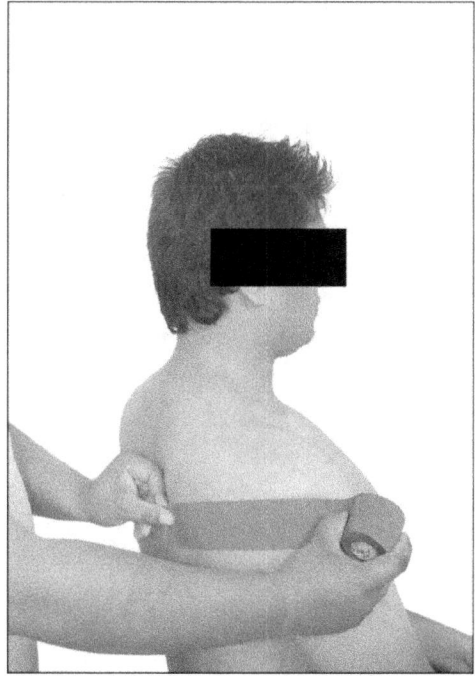

Figure 2.29: Measuring the tape.

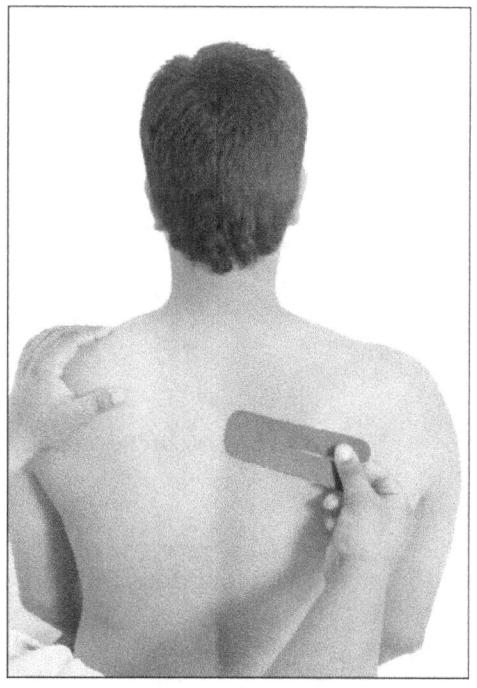

Figure 2.30: Application of base.

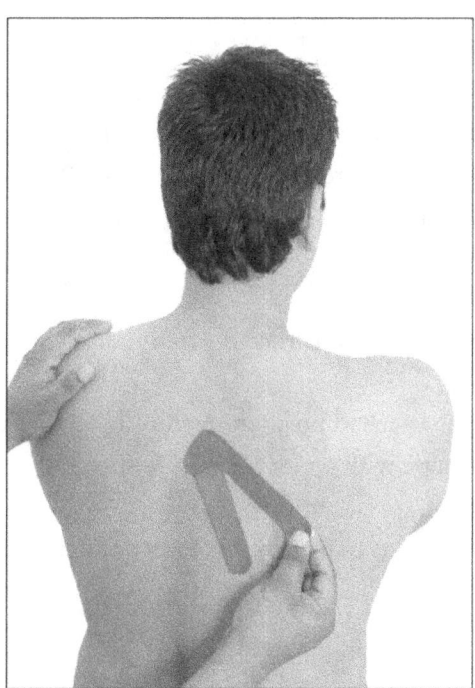

Figure 2.31: Application of tail.

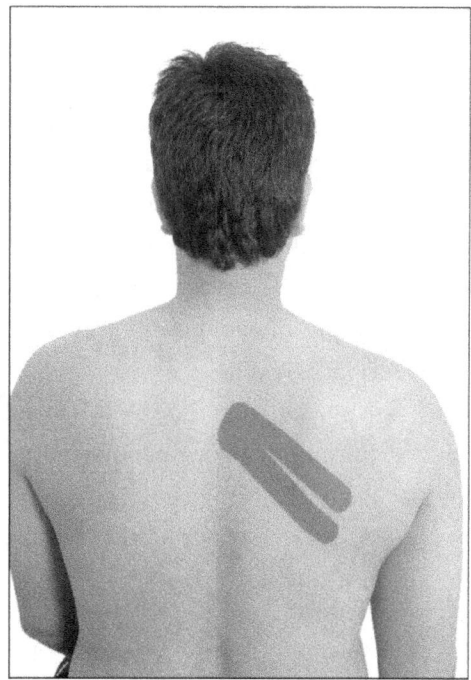

Figure 2.32: Final application.

# Pectoralis Minor

**Technique Used**: Muscle tonus down Technique.

**Muscle**: Pectoralis minor[40,92.]

**Origin**:

- Ribs 3-5.

**Insertion**:

- Coracoid process of the scapula.

**Function**:

- It moves scapula forward, medial, and downward.

**Innervations**: Medial Pectoral Nerve.

**Subject Position**: Subject sitting in relaxed comfortable position.

**Therapist Position**: Therapist standing behind the subject.

**Strip:** Y strip is used.

**Procedure:**

- Follow the basic steps for muscle taping.
- Measuring the tape:  The subject is asked to retract the shoulders with extension of arm, the tape is measured from 5th rib on mid clavicular line to corocoid process (Fig: 2.33).
- Select the required strip design, for large muscle bulk, use "I" strip and in small muscle generally the "Y" strip.
- The corners of the tapes are rounded off.
- Application of base: Apply the base with no stretch, distal to corocoid process of scapula (Fig: 2.34).
- Application of the tail: When subject's muscle is in stretched position, therapist stabilizes the base with one hand and applies the rest of the tape with paper off or 10% stretch (Fig: 2.35).
- At the end of application rub the tape until the warmth is felt, this is necessary to activate the glue.

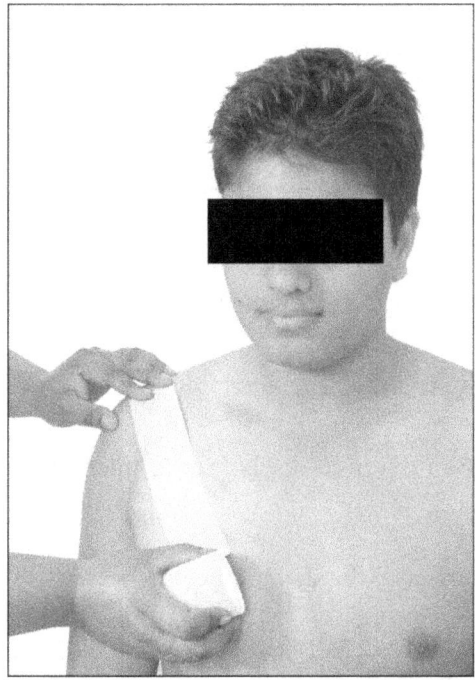

Figure 2.33: Measuring the tape.

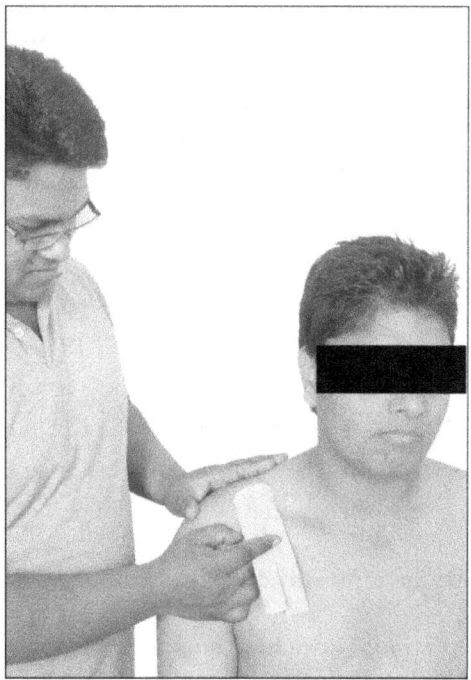

Figure 2.34: Application of base.

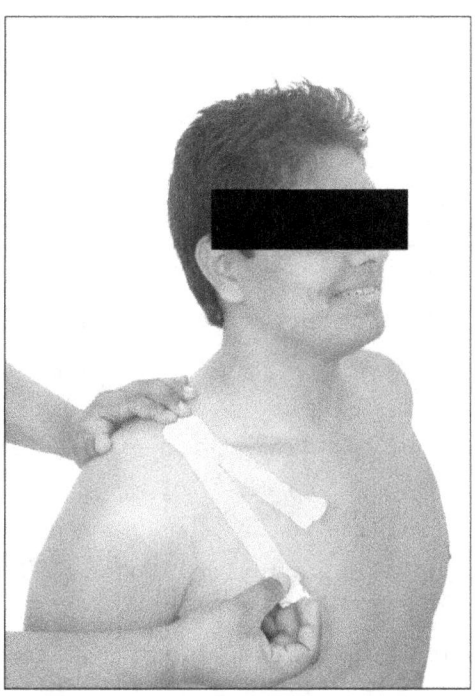

Figure 2.35: Application of tail.

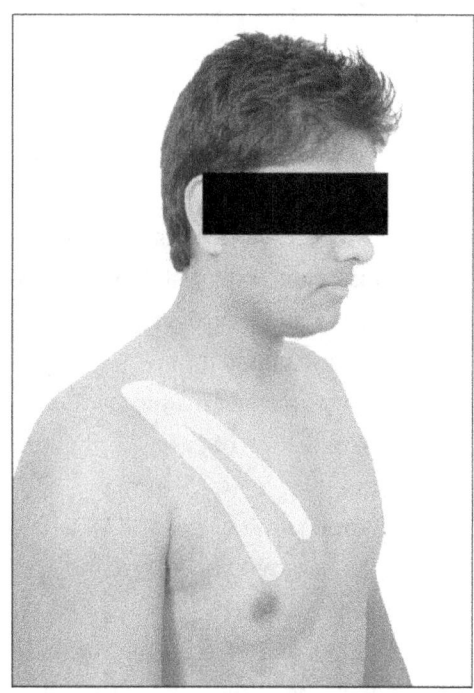

Figure 2.36: Final application.

# Deltoid

**Technique used**: Muscle tonus down Technique.

**Muscle**: Deltoid[14].

**Origin**: The deltoid originates in three distinct sets of fibers:

- The anterior fibers arise from the anterior border and upper surface of the lateral third of the clavicle;
- Lateral or acromial fibers arise from the superior surface of the acromion process. They are commonly called lateral deltoid;
- Posterior or spinal fibers arise from the lower lip of the posterior border of the spine of the scapula.

**Insertion**: It inserts into the deltoid tuberosity on the lateral surface of the shaft of the humerus.

**Innervation**: The deltoid muscle is innervated by the axillary nerve.

**Function**: The major function of the deltoid muscle is abduction of the arm.

**Subject position**: Subject sitting in relaxed comfortable position.

**Therapist position**: Therapist standing behind the subject.

**Strip**: I-strip is used.

**Procedure:**

- Follow the basic steps for muscle taping.
- Measuring the tape: The subject is asked to do horizontal adduction of the shoulder so as to put deltoid muscle in a stretched position, the tape is measured from midpoint of clavicle to 2cm distal to insertion of deltoid muscle (Fig: 2.37).
- Select the required strip design, for large muscle bulk, use two "I" strip and in small muscle generally the "Y" strip.
- The corners of the tapes are rounded off.
- Application of base: Apply the base with no stretch just 2 cm distal to the insertion while the subject is in neutral position or the resting position (Fig: 2.38).
- Application of the tail: When subject's muscle is in stretched position, therapist stablises the base with one hand and applies the rest of the tape with paper off or 10% stretch (Fig: 2.39, Fig 2.41).
- At the end of application rub the tape until the warmth is felt, this is necessary to activate the glue.

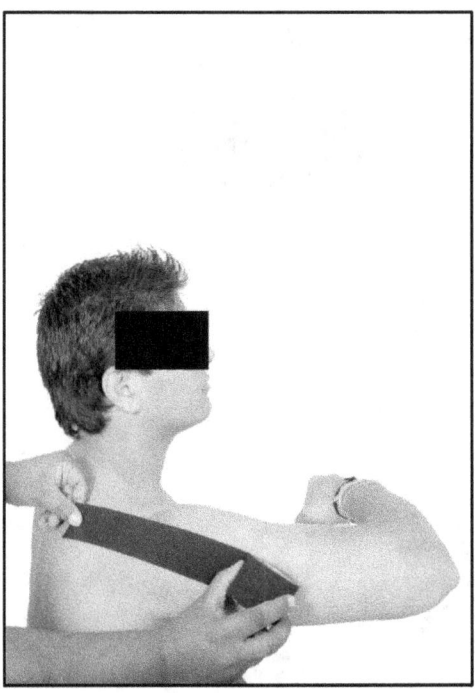

Figure 2.37: Measuring the tape.

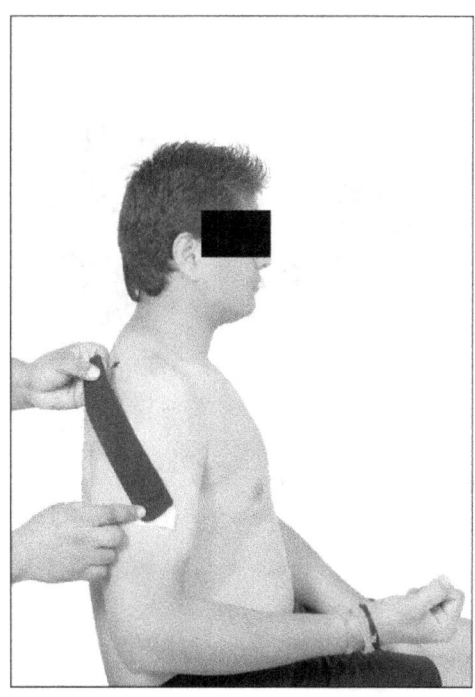

Figure 2.38: Application of base.

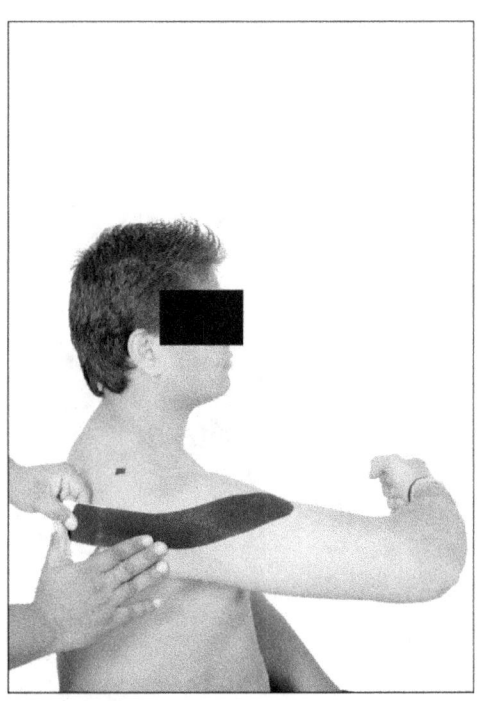

Figure 2.39: Application of tail.

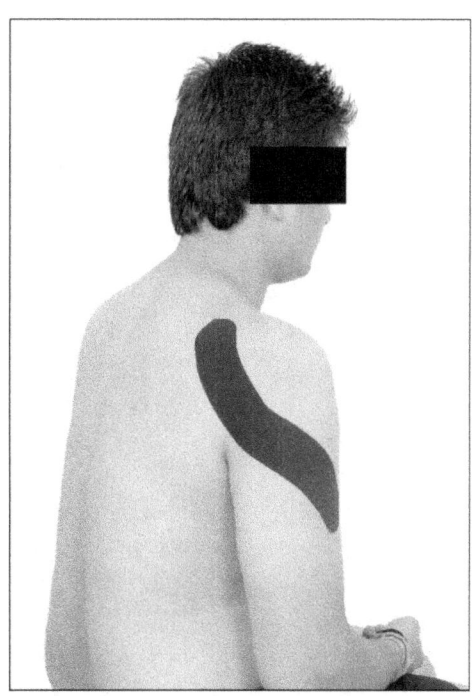

Figure 2.40: Final application.

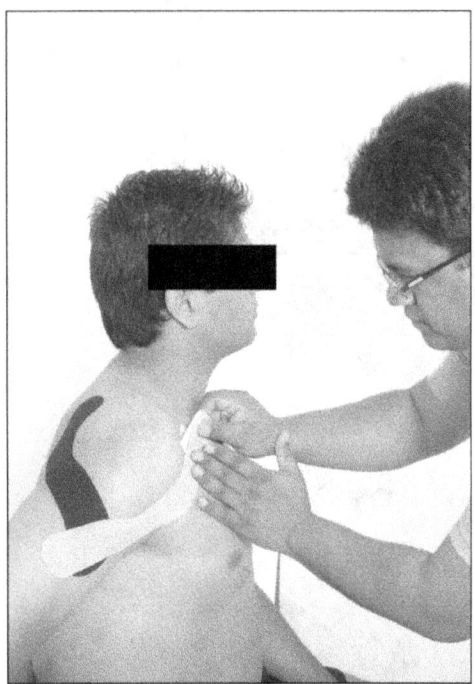

Figure 2.41: Application of tail.

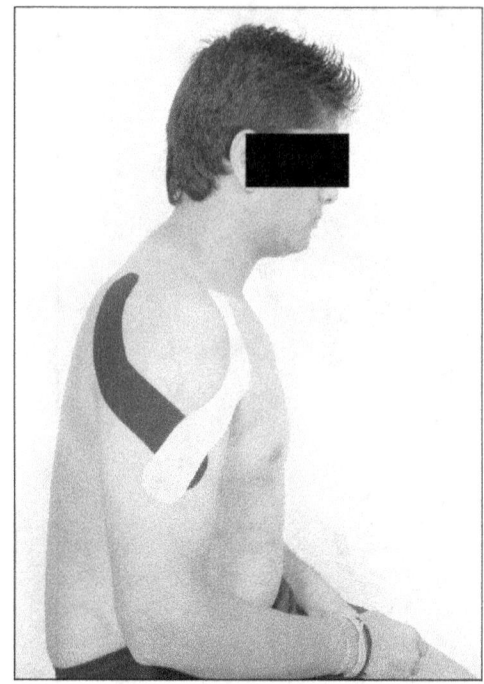

Figure 2.42: Final application.

# Biceps Brachii

**Technique Used**: Muscle tonus down Technique.

**Muscle**: Biceps Brachii[72,78,81].

**Origin**:

- The short head of the muscle originates from the coracoid process ,
- The long head originates as a tendon from the supraglenoid tubercle of the scapula.

 **Insertion**: The long and short heads converge to form a single tendon, which inserts onto the radial tuberosity.

**Function**:

- Flexor of the forearm at the elbow joint;
- The most powerful Supinator of the forearm when the elbow joint is flexed;
- The muscle can also flex the Glenohumeral joint.

**Innervations**: The Musculocutaneous nerve.

**Subject Position**: Subject sitting in relaxed comfortable position.

**Therapist Position**: Therapist standing behind the subject.

**Strip:** Y strip is used.

**Procedure:**

- Follow the basic steps for muscle taping.
- Measuring the tape:  The subject is asked to extend the arm, the tape is measured from the radial tuberosity to 2 cm proximal to the coracoid process (Fig: 2.43).
- Select the required strip design, for large muscle bulk, use "I" strip and in small muscle generally the "Y" strip.
- The corners of the tapes are rounded off.
- Application of base: Apply the base with no stretch just on anterior surface of upper limb, just below the radial tuberosity (Fig: 2.44).
- Application of the tail: When subject's muscle is in stretched position, therapist stabilizes the base with one hand and applies the rest of the tape with paper off or 10% stretch (Fig: 2.45).
- At the end of application rub the tape until the warmth is felt, this is necessary to activate the glue.

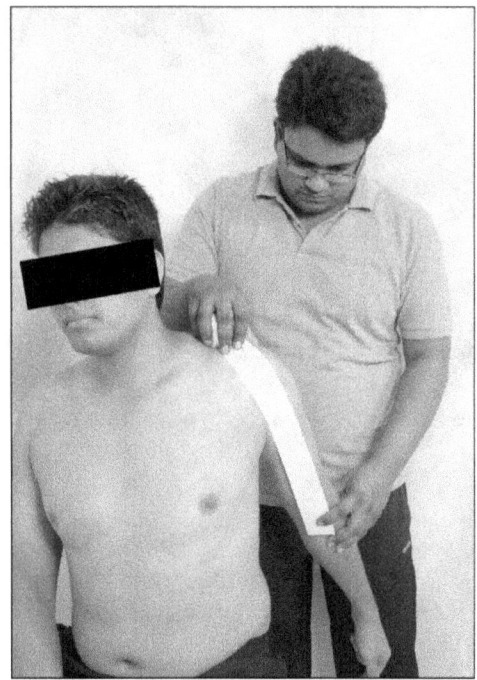

Figure 2.43: Measuring the tape.

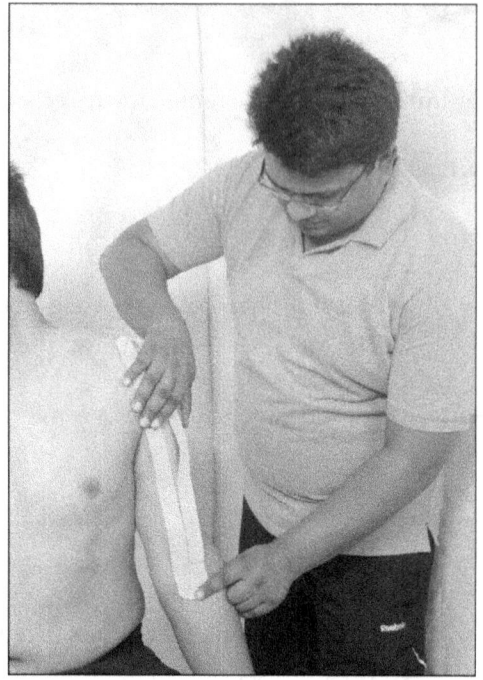

Figure 2.44: Application of base.

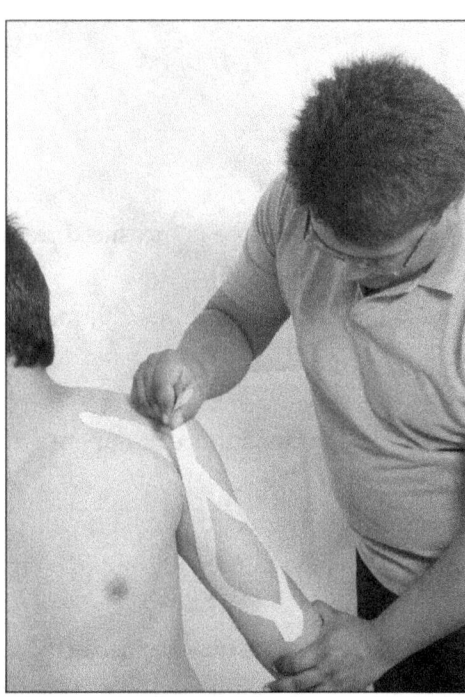

Figure 2.45: Application of tail.

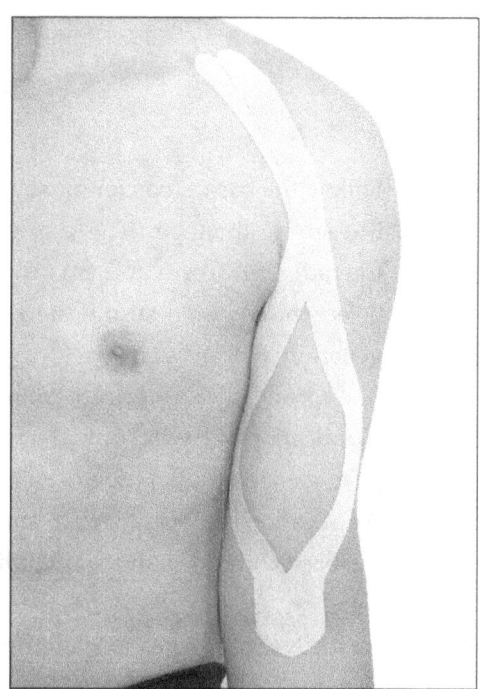

Figure 2.46: Final application.

# Triceps

**Technique used**: Muscle tonus down Technique.

**Muscle**: Triceps[37,73].

**Origin:**

- Long head - infraglenoid tubercle of the scapula,
- Lateral head - upper half of the posterior surface of the shaft of the humerus, and the upper part of the lateral intermuscular septum,
- Medial head - posterior shaft of humerus, distal to radial groove and both the medial and lateral intermuscular septum (deep to the long & lateral heads).

**Insertion:**

- Posterior surface of the olecranon process of the ulna,
- Deep fascia of the antebrachium.

**Innervation**: Radial nerve, C6, C7.

**Function:**

- Long - adducts the arm, extends at the shoulder, and a little elbow flexion;
- Lateral and Medial head- extends the forearm at the elbow.

**Subject position**: Subject sitting in relaxed comfortable position.

**Therapist position**: Therapist standing at the affected side of the subject.

**Strip**: Y strip is used.

**Procedure:**

- Follow the basic steps for muscle taping.
- Measuring the tape: The subject is asked to flex the shoulder and elbow, the tape is measured 2 cm distal to the olecronon process of the ulna to the inferior of apex of axilla (Fig: 2.47).
- Select the required strip design, for large muscle bulk, use two "I" strip and in small muscle generally the "Y" strip.
- The corners of the tapes are rounded off.
- Application of base: Apply the base with no stretch just 2cm proximal to the origin from infraglenoid tubercle while the subject is in neutral position or the resting position (Fig: 2.48).
- Application of the tail: When subject's muscle is in stretched position, therapist stablises the base with one hand and applies the rest of the tape with paper off or 10% stretch (Fig: 2.49).
- At the end of application rub the tape until the warmth is felt, this is necessary to activate the glue.

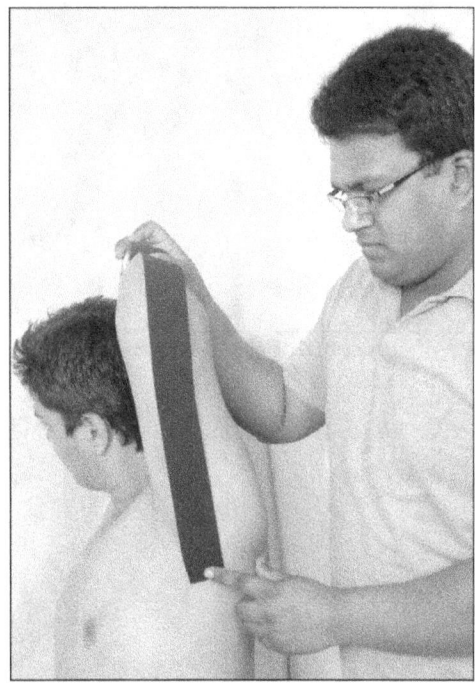

Figure 2.47: Measuring the tape.

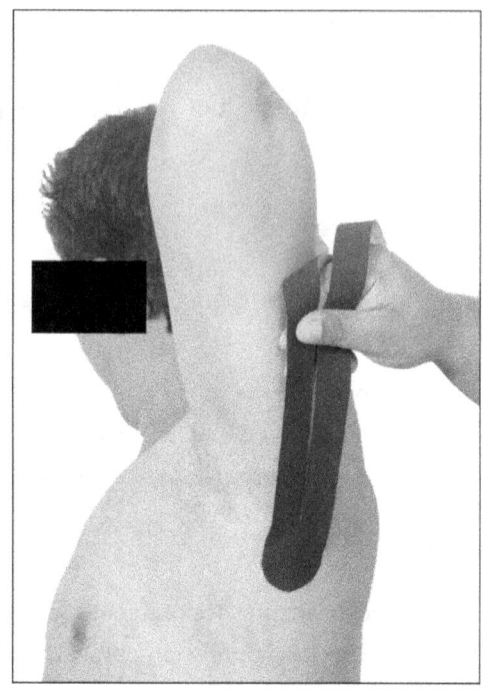

Figure 2.48: Application of base.

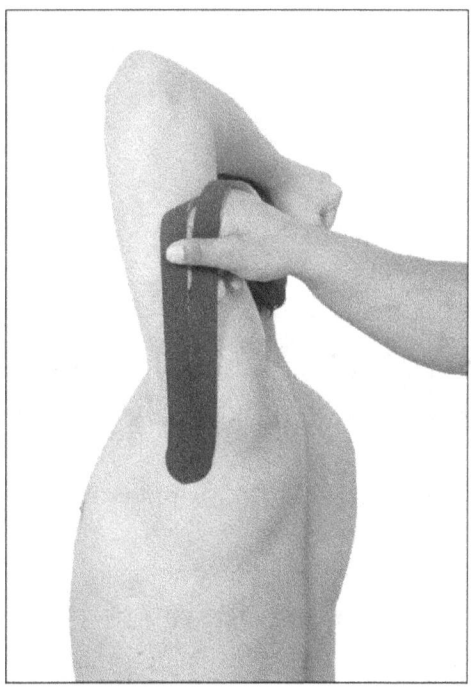

Figure 2.49: Application of tail.

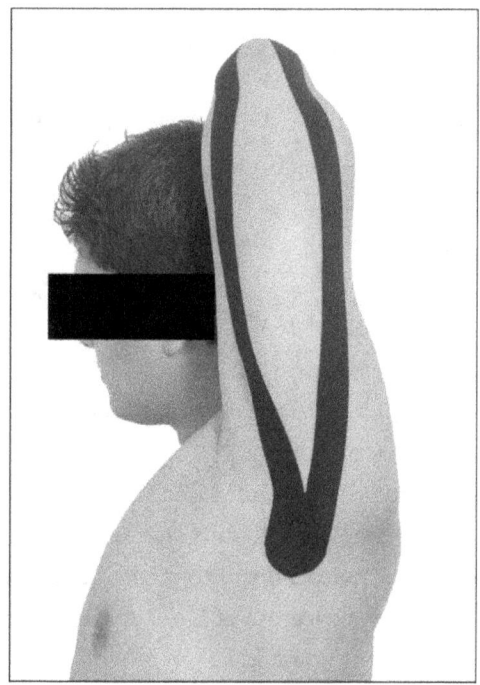

Figure 2.50: Final application.

## Rectus Femoris

**Technique used**: Muscle tonus up Technique.

**Muscle:** Rectus femoris[3,34].

**Origin:**

- Anterior head: anterior inferior iliac spine (AIIS),
- Posterior head: ilium just above the acetabulum.

**Insertion:**

- Common quadriceps tendon into patella,
- Tibial tuberosity via patellar ligament.

**Innervation:** Branches of femoral nerve, [L2].

**Function:**

- Extends knee;
- Flexes hip.

**Subject's position**: Subject lying supine with affected leg handing out of the couch.

**Therapist position**: Therapist sitting to the affected side of the subject's leg.

**Strip**: Y and I combination tape is used.

**Procedure:**

- Follow the basic steps for muscle taping.
- Measuring the tape: The subject is in supine lying with the affected leg hanging out of the couch, the rectus femoris is in stretch position with the knee in flexion, and the tape is measured from anterior inferior iliac spine to 2cm distal to tibial tuberosity (Fig: 2.51).
- Select the required strip design, for large muscle bulk, use "I" strip and just cut it into "Y" just above the patella.
- The corners of the tapes are rounded off.
- Application of base: Apply the base with no stretch just 2 cm proximal to the AIIS (Fig: 2.52).
- Application of the tail: When subject's muscle is in stretched position, therapist stablises the base with one hand and applies the rest of the tape with paper off or 10% stretch (Fig: 2.53).
- At the end of application rub the tape until the warmth is felt, this is necessary to activate the glue.

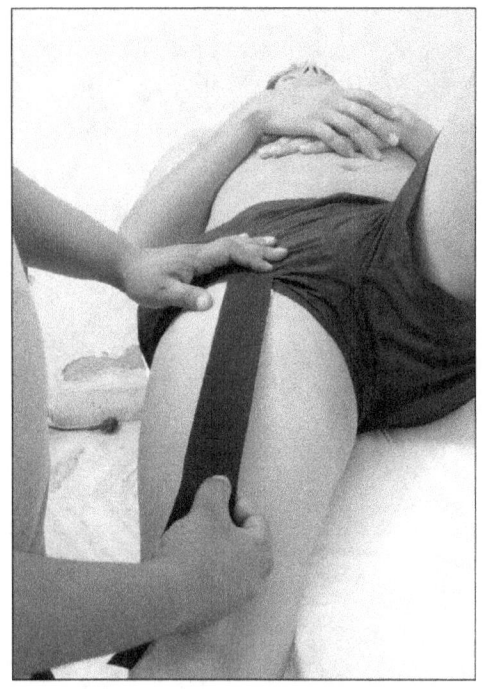

Figure 2.51: Measuring the tape.

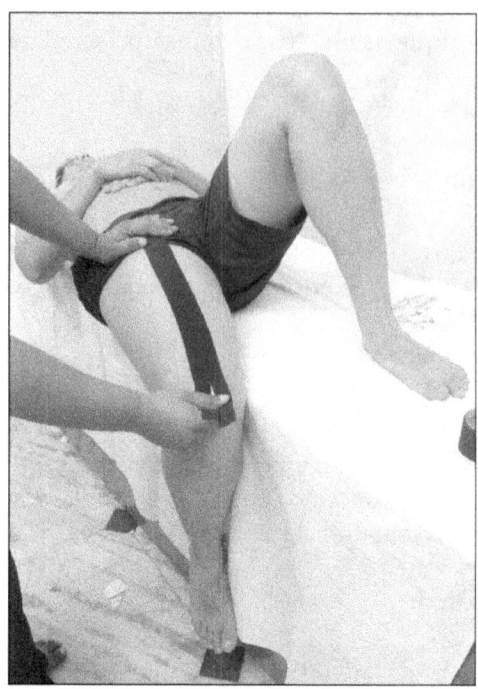

Figure 2.52: Application of base.

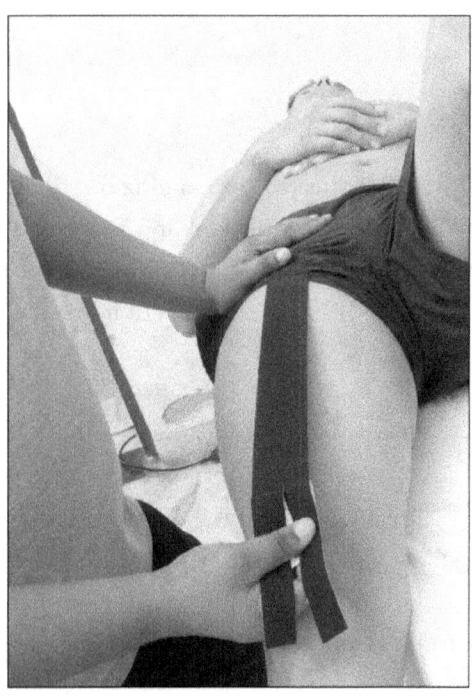

Figure 2.53: Application of tail.

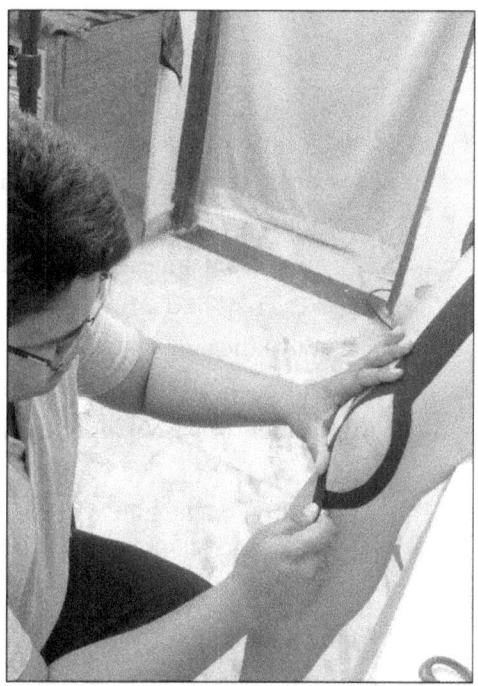

Figure 2.54: Final application.

# Biceps Femoris

**Technique used**: Muscle tonus down Technique.

**Muscle:** Biceps Femoris[72].

**Origin:**

- Long head: Ischial Tuberosity,
- Short head: lateral lip of linea aspera and the lateral inter-muscular septum.

**Insertion:**

- Head of Fibula;
- To the lateral Tibial Condyle.

**Innervation:**

- Long head - Tibial nerve, L5,S1,2,
- Short head - Common Peroneal Nerve, L5, S1.

**Function:**

- Flexor at the knee (mainly short head),
- Laterally rotates thigh if flexed at the knee,
- Extends hip (long head).

**Subject's position**: Subject standing in comfortable position.

**Therapist position**: Therapist sitting at the affected side of subject leg.

**Strip:** I shaped tape is used.

**Procedure:**

- Follow the basic steps for muscle taping.
- Measuring the tape: The subject is asked to do forward trunk flexion, the tape is measured from head of fibula to ischial tuberosity (Fig: 2.55).
- Select the required strip design, for large muscle bulk, use "I" strip and just cut it into "Y" just above the patella.
- The corners of the tapes are rounded off.
- Application of base: Apply the base with no stretch just 2 cm distal to head of fibula while the subject is standing straight (Fig: 2.56).
- Application of the tail: When subject's muscle is in stretched position, therapist stablises the base with one hand and applies the rest of the tape with paper off or 10% stretch (Fig: 2.57).
- At the end of application rub the tape until the warmth is felt, this is necessary to activate the glue.

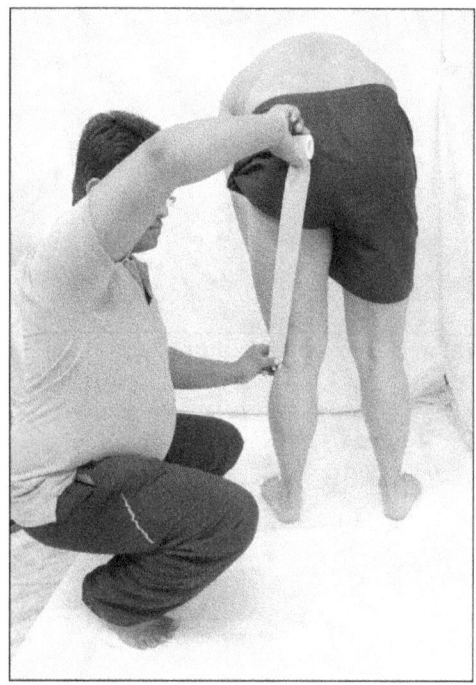

Figure 2.55: Measuring the tape.

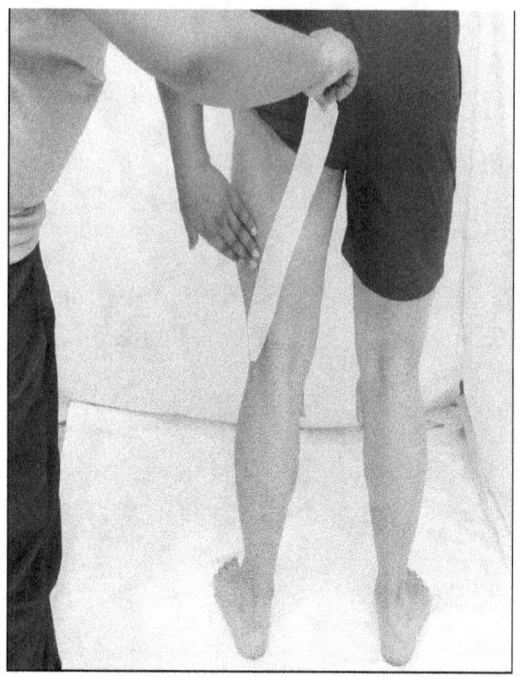

Figure 2.56: Application of base.

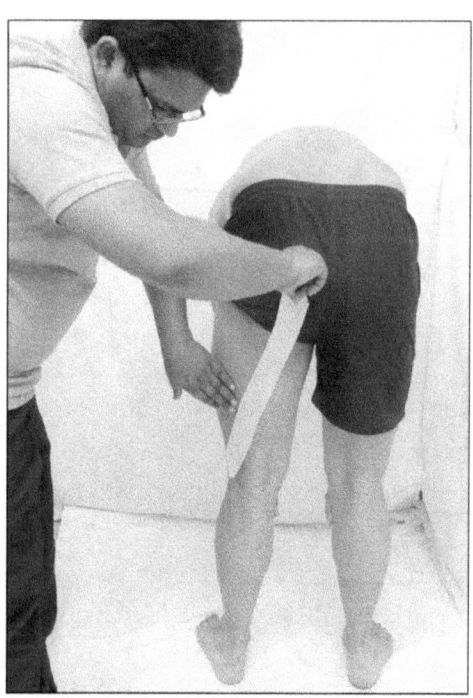

Figure 2.57: Application of tail.

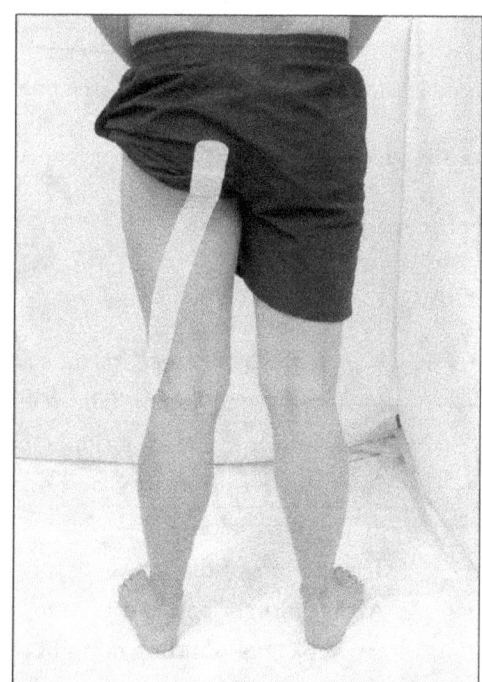

Figure 2.58: Final application.

# Semimembranosus

**Technique used:** Muscle tonus down Technique.

**Muscle:** Semimembranosus.

**Origin:**

- Ischial tuberosity.

**Insertion:**

- Posterior medial aspect of medial tibial condyle,
- Fibers join to form most of oblique popliteal ligament.

**Function:**

- Flexes knee,
- Extends hip,
- Medially rotates tibia,
- Pulls medial meniscus posterior during flexion.

**Innervation:** Tibial nerve of sciatic bundle, L5, S1, S2.

**Subject's position:** Standing in a comfortable position.

**Therapist position:** Standing behind the subject.

**Strip:** I shaped tape is used.

**Procedure:**

- Follow the basic steps for muscle taping.
- Measuring the tape: The subject is asked to bend forward (forward flexion of trunk), the tape is measured from medial tibial condyle to ischial tuberosity (Fig: 2.59).
- Select the required strip design, for large muscle bulk, use "I" strip and in small muscle generally the "Y" strip.
- The corners of the tapes are rounded off.
- Application of base: Apply the base with no stretch on the posterior medial aspect of medial tibial condyle (Fig: 2.60).
- Application of the tail: When subject's muscle is in stretched position, therapist stabilizes the base with one hand and applies the rest of the tape with paper off or 10% stretch (Fig: 2.61).
- At the end of application rub the tape until the warmth is felt, this is necessary to activate the glue.

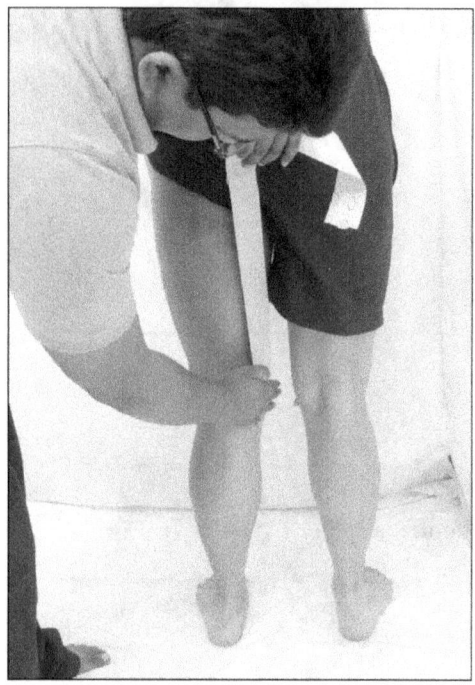

Figure 2.59: Measuring the tape.

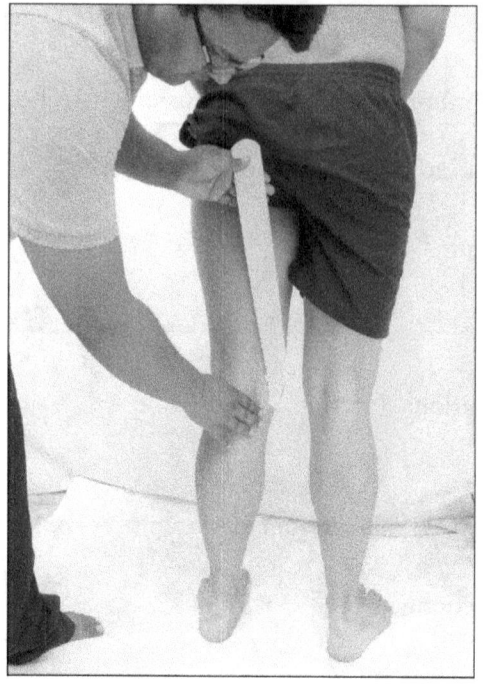

Figure 2.60: Application of base.

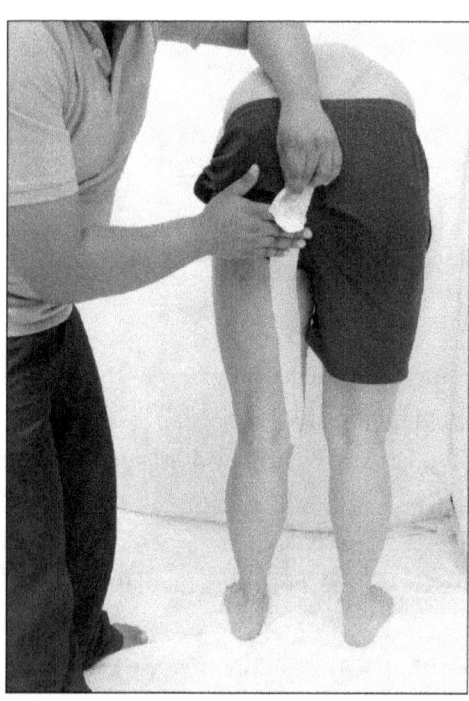

Figure 2.61: Application of tail.

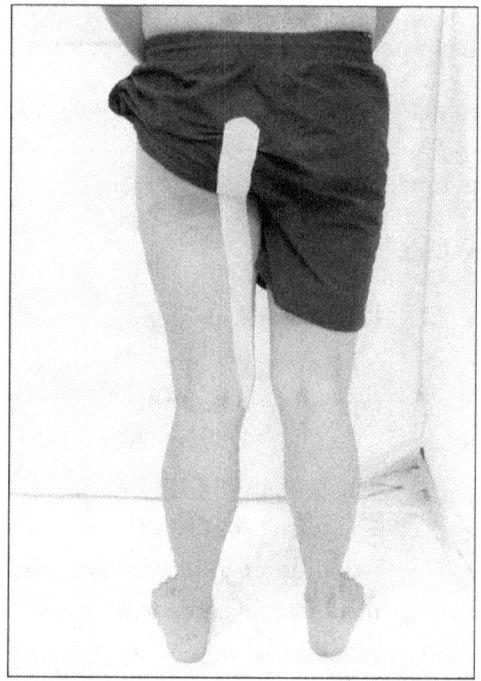

Figure 2.62: Final application.

# Adductor Magnus

**Technique used:** Muscle tonus down Technique.

**Muscle:** Adductor magnus.

**Origin:**

- Anterior fibers: inferior pubic ramus,
- Oblique fibers: ischial ramus,
- Posterior fibers: ischial tuberosity.

**Insertion:**

- Proximal 1/3 of linea aspera,
- Adductor tubercle.

**Function:**

- Adducts the thigh,
- Posterior fibers also extend and laterally rotate thigh.

**Innervation:**

- Anterior fibers: Obturator nerve, L2,3,4,
- Posterior fibers: Tibial nerve of sciatic bundle, L4,5.

**Subject's position:** Lying supine on the couch.

**Therapist position:** Standing on the affected side of the limb.

**Strip**: I shaped tape is used.

**Procedure:**

- Follow the basic steps for muscle taping.
- Measuring the tape:  The subject is asked to abduct the hip joint and the tape is measured from adductor tubercle just above the medial condyle of the femur to the 2 cm proximal to superior part on inner thigh (Fig: 2.63).
- Select the required strip design, for large muscle bulk, use "I" strip and in small muscle generally the "Y" strip.
- The corners of the tapes are rounded off.
- Application of base: Apply the base with no stretch just 2cm distal to the adductor tubercle while the subject is in neutral position or the resting position (Fig: 2.64).
- Application of the tail: When subject's muscle is in stretched position, therapist stablises the base with one hand and applies the rest of the tape with paper off or 10% stretch (Fig: 2.65).
- At the end of application rub the tape until the warmth is felt, this is necessary to activate the glue.

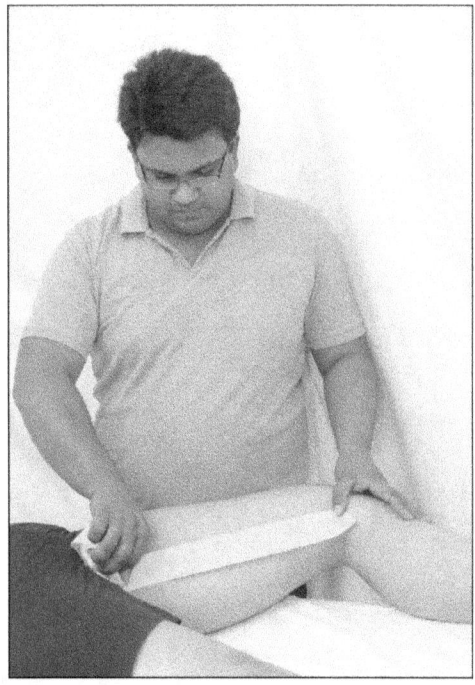

Figure 2.63: Measuring the tape.

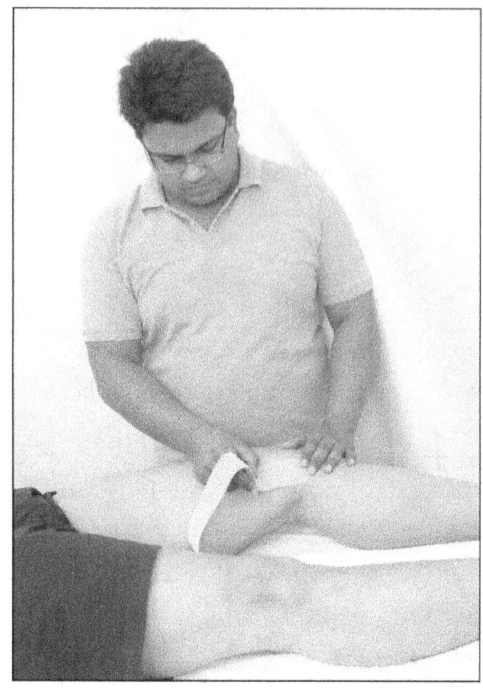

Figure 2.64: Application of base.

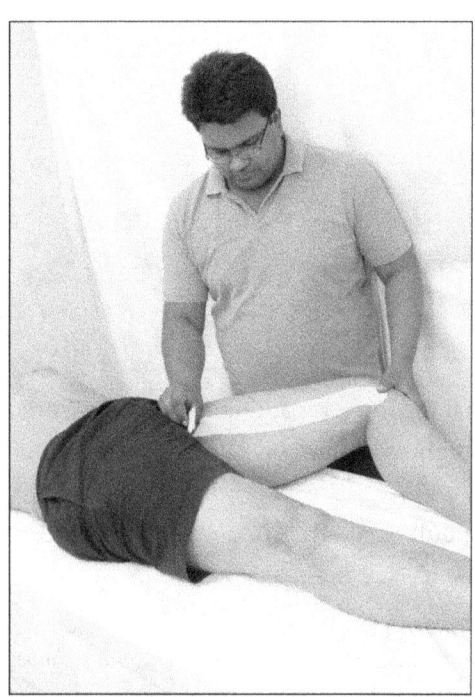

Figure 2.65: Application of tail.

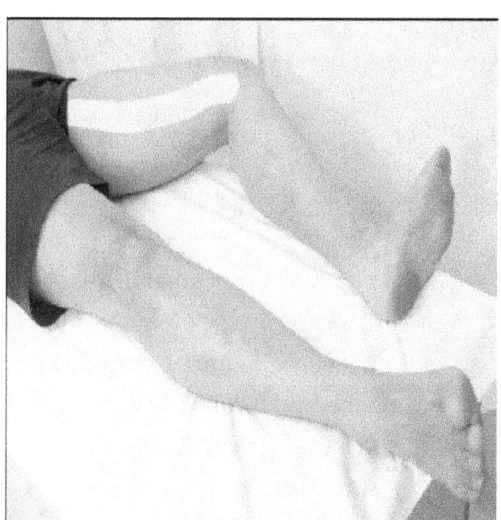

Figure 2.66: Final application.

# Tibialis Anterior

**Technique used:** Muscle tonus up Technique.

**.Muscle:** Tibialis Anterior[1,9].

**Origin:**

- Lateral tibial condyle,
- Proximal 2/3 of anteriolateral surface of tibia,
- Interosseous membrane,
- Anterior intermuscular septum & crural fascia.

**Insertion:**

- Medial &  plantar surface of base of 1st metatarsal,
- Medial & plantar surface of the cuneiform.

**Function:**

- Strongest dorsiflexor of ankle,
- Inverts & adducts the foot.

**Innervation:** Deep Peroneal Nerve, L4, L5, S1.

**Subject's position:** Supine Lying.

**Therapist position:** Therapist stands at the side of the subject

**Strip:**I shaped tape is used.

**Procedure:**

- Follow the basic steps for muscle taping.
- Measuring the tape:  The subject is asked to planter flex and everts the foot, the tape is measured from lateral tibial condyle to approx. 2 cm distal to base of 1st metatarsals (Fig: 2.67).
- Select the required strip design, for large muscle bulk, use "I" strip and in small muscle generally the "Y" strip.
- The corners of the tapes are rounded off.
- Application of base: Apply the base with no stretch just above the lateral tibial condyle (Fig: 2.68).
- Application of the tail: When subject's muscle is in stretched position, therapist stabilizes the base with one hand and applies the rest of the tape with paper off or 10% stretch (Fig: 2.69).
- At the end of application rub the tape until the warmth is felt, this is necessary to activate the glue.

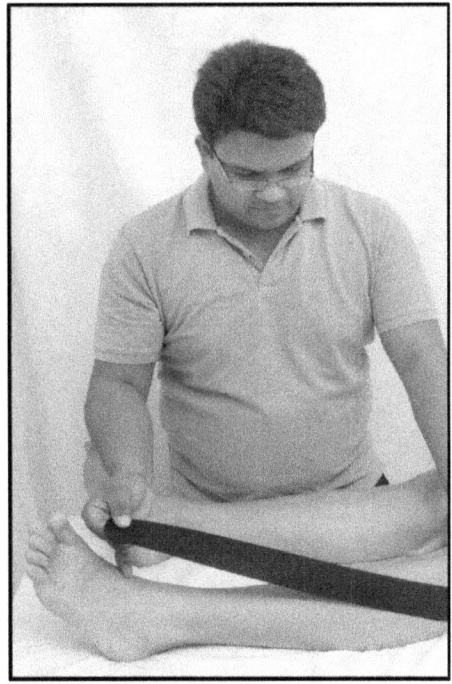

Figure 2.67: Measuring the tape.

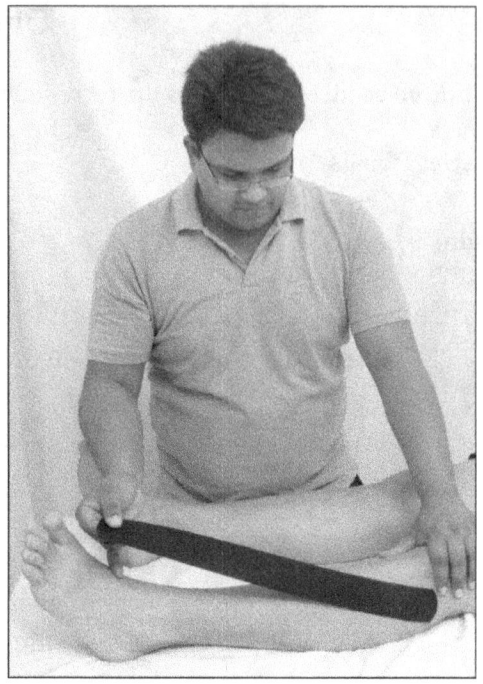

Figure 2.68: Application of base.

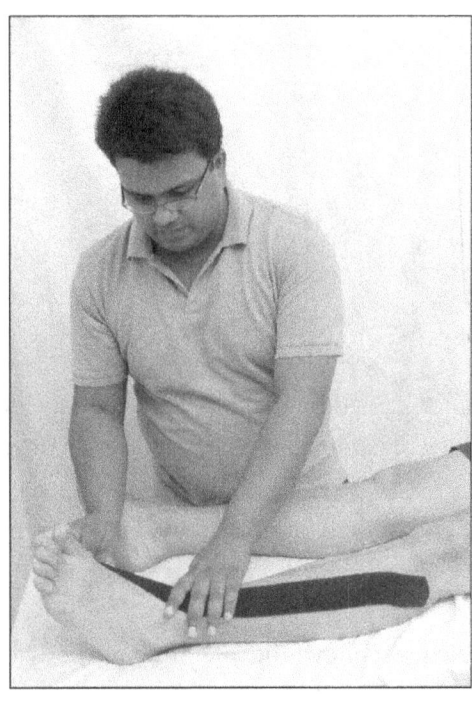

Figure 2.69: Application of tail.

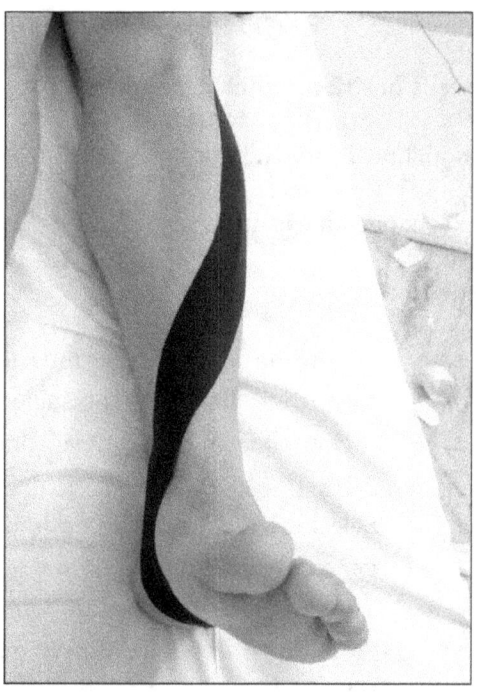

Figure 2.70: Final application.

# Gastrosoleus (Tricpes Surae)

**Technique used:** Muscle tonus down Technique.

**Muscle**: Gastrocnemius and Soleus[45].

**Origin:**

- Gastrocnemius -Lateral head originates from the lateral condyle of the femur, while the medial head originates from the medial condyle of the femur.
- Soleus muscle - Fibers originate from each side of the anterior aponeurosis, and from the posterior surfaces of the head of the fibula and its upper quarter, as well as the middle third of the medial border of the tibia.

**Insertion:**

- The posterior aponeurosis and median septum join in the lower quarter of the muscle and then join with the anterior aponeuroses of the gastrocnemius muscles to form the calcaneal tendon or Achilles tendon and inserts onto the posterior surface of the calcaneum.

**Innervation:** The triceps surae is innervated by the tibial nerve.

**Function:**

- Planter flexion of the ankle complex.

**Subject's position:** Subject lying prone with foot at edge of the couch.

**Therapist position**: Therapist standing at foot end of the couch.

**Strip:** I and Y both shaped strips are used.

**Procedure:**

- Follow the basic steps for muscle taping.
- Measuring the tape:  The subject is asked to dorsiflex the ankle and 2 tapes are measured from 2 cm distal to insertion of Achilles tendon, to the midpoint of posterior of knee joint (Fig: 2.71).
- Select the required strip design, for large muscle bulk, use "I" strip and in small muscle generally the "Y" strip.
- The corners of the tapes are rounded off.
- Application of base: Apply the base with no stretch just on planter surface of calcaneum while the ankle is in neutral position (Fig: 2.72).
- Application of the tail: When subject's muscle is in stretched position, therapist stablises the base with one hand and applies the rest of the tape with paper off or 10% stretch (Fig: 2.73).
- At the end of application rub the tape until the warmth is felt, this is necessary to activate the glue.

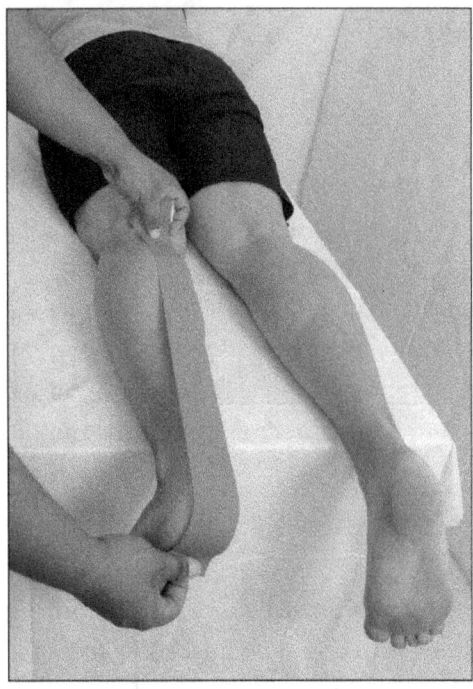

Figure 2.71: Measuring the tape.

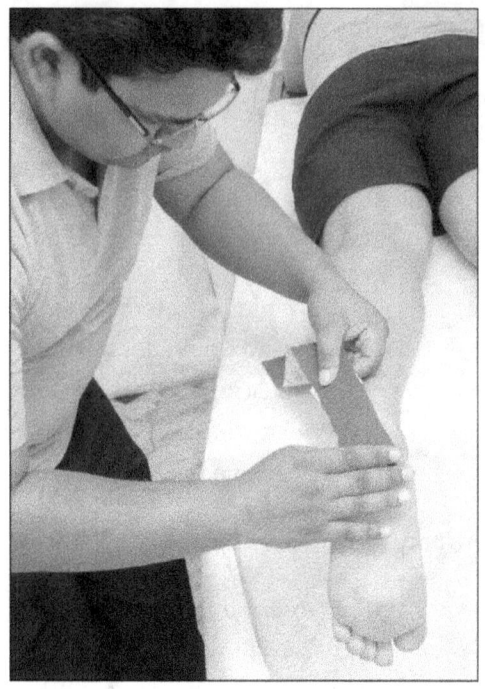

Figure 2.72: Application of base.

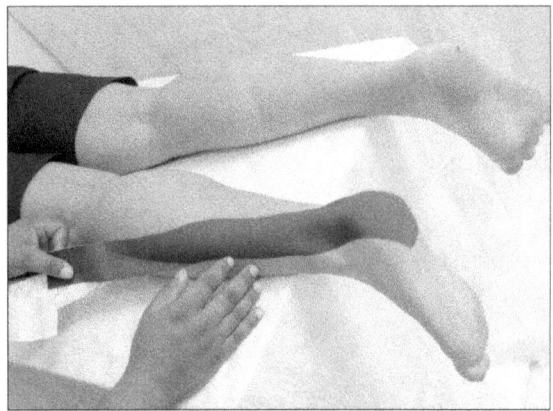
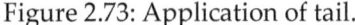

Figure 2.73: Application of tail.

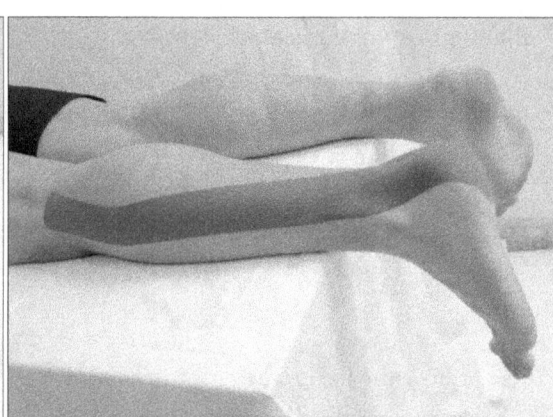

Figure 2.74: Final application.

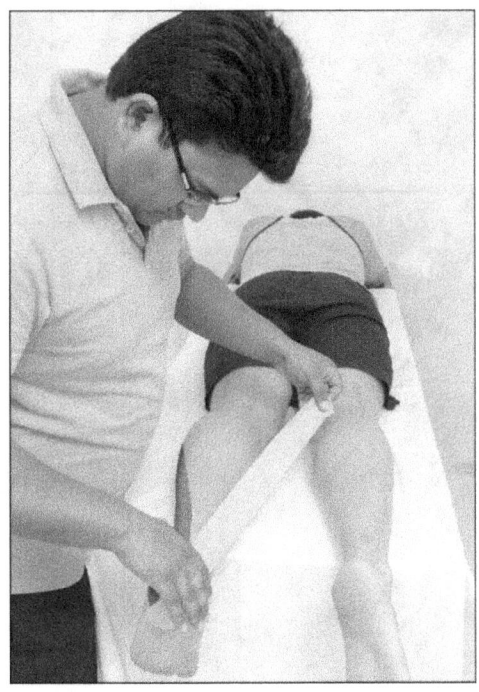

Figure 2.75: Application of tail.

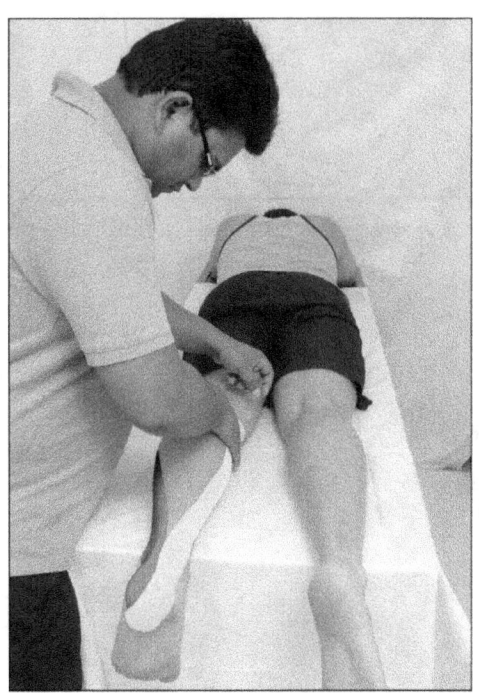

Figure 2.76: Application of tail.

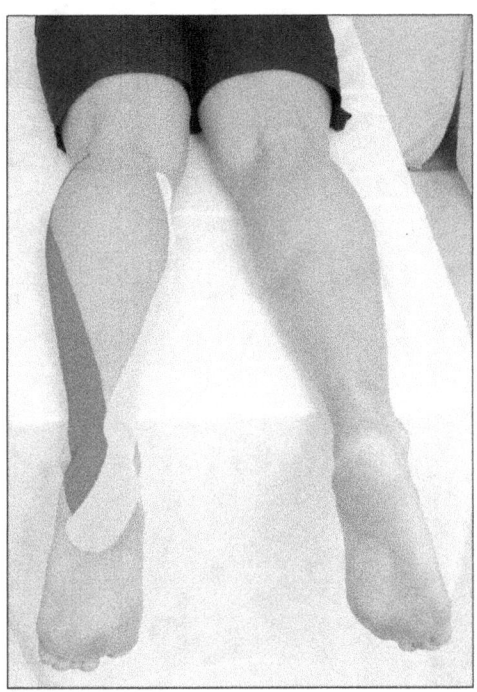

Figure 2.77: Final application.

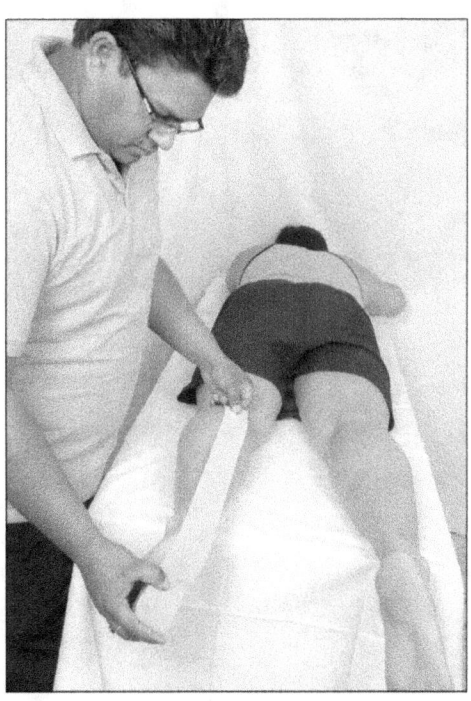

Figure 2.78: Measuring the tape for soleus.

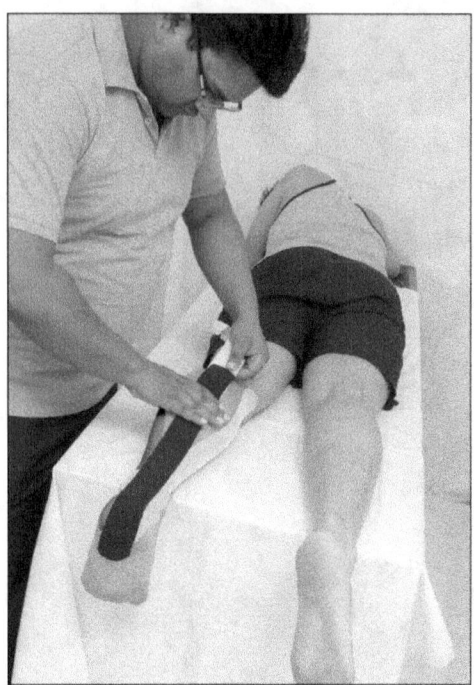

Figure 2.79: Application of tail.

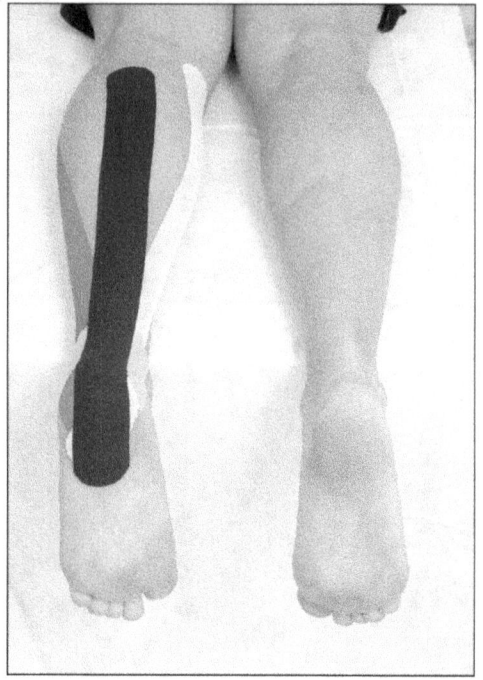

Figure 2.80: Final application.

# Tibialis Posterior

**Technique Used**: Muscle tonus up Technique.

.**Muscle**: Tibialis posterior[43].

**Origin**:

- Interosseous membrane,
- Posteromedial surface of the fibula,
- Posterolateral surface of the tibia

**Insertion**:

- Tuberosity of the navicular,
- Medial cuneiform,
- Metatarsals 2-4.

**Function**:

- Plantar flexes the foot;
- Inverts the foot.

**Innervations:** Tibial nerve.

**Subject Position**: Subject lying prone on the couch with foot out of the couch.

**Therapist Position**: Therapist standing at the foot end of the couch.

**Strip:** Y strip is used.

**Procedure:**

- Follow the basic steps for muscle taping.
- Measuring the tape: The subject is asked to dorsiflex the ankle and tape is measured from head of fibula to the 4th metatarsal (Fig: 2.81).
- Select the required strip design, for large muscle bulk, use "I" strip and in small muscle generally the "Y" strip.
- The corners of the tapes are rounded off.
- Application of base: Apply one tail of base with no stretch on the posterior medial aspect of the head of fibula and one at 2-3 cm medially from head of fibula towards tibia (Fig: 2.82).
- Application of the tail: When subject's muscle is in stretched position, therapist stabilizes the base with one hand and applies the rest of the tape with paper off or 10% stretch (Fig: 2.83).
- At the end of application rub the tape until the warmth is felt, this is necessary to activate the glue.

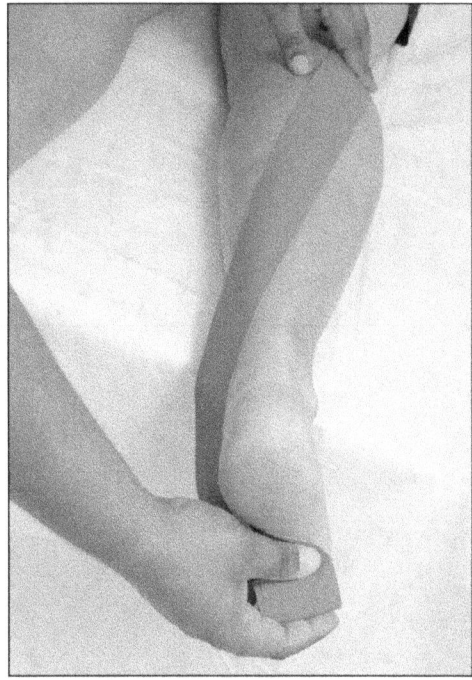

Figure 2.81: Measuring the tape.

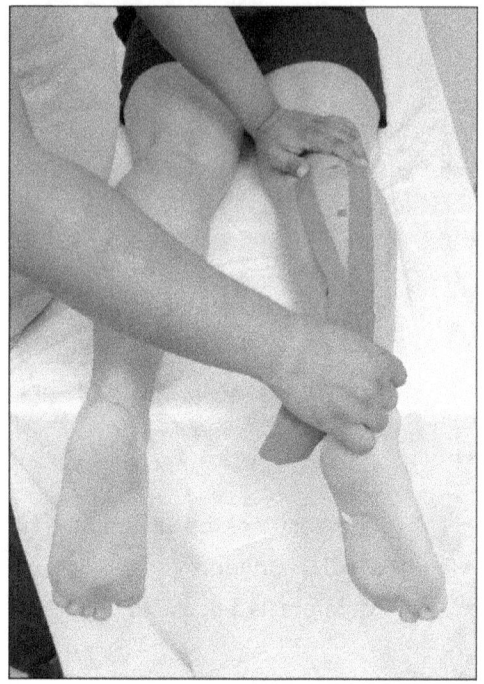

Figure 2.82: Application of base.

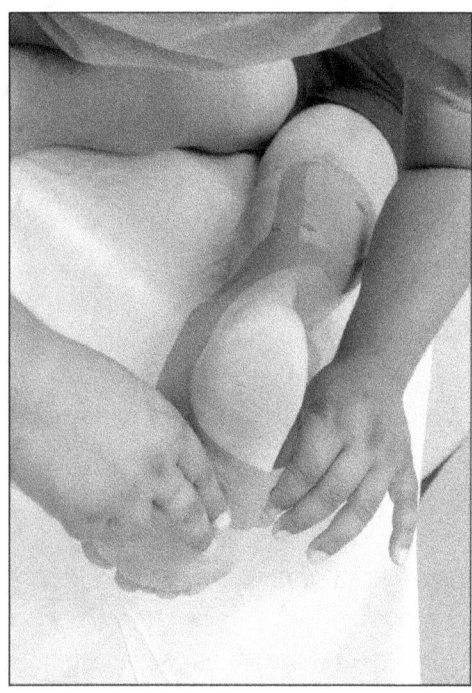

Figure 2.83: Application of tail.

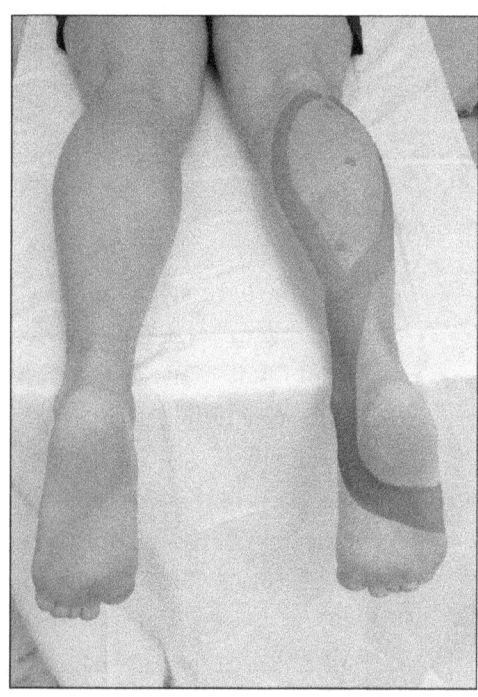

Figure 2.84: Final application.

# Extensor Hallucis Longus

**Technique used:** Muscle tonus down Technique.

**Muscle:** Extensor Hallucis Longus.

**Origin:**

- Medial aspect of the fibula,
- Interosseous membrane,
- Crural fascia.

**Insertion:** Dorsal surface of base of proximal and distal phalanx of hallux.

**Innervation:** Deep Peroneal nerve, L4, L5, S1.

**Function:**

- Extends distal phalanx of big toe,
- Weak dorsiflexor of ankle,
- Weak invertor and adductor of foot.

**Subject's position:** Subject lying supine with foot at edge of the couch.

**Therapist position:** Therapist standing at foot end of the couch.

**Strip:** I shaped tape is used.

**Procedure:**

- Follow the basic steps for muscle taping.
- Measuring the tape: The subject is asked to flex the great toe with plantar flexion of the ankle, the tape is measured from the tip of great toe to 2 cm below the proximal condyle of tibia (Fig: 2.8)5.
- Select the required strip design, for large muscle bulk, use "I" strip and in small muscle generally the "Y" strip.
- The corners of the tapes are rounded off.
- Application of base: Apply the base with no stretch just on dorsal surface of the distal phalanx of the great toe while the toe and ankle are in neutral position (Fig: 2.86).
- Application of the tail: When subject's muscle is in stretched position, therapist stablises the base with one hand and applies the rest of the tape with paper off or 10% stretch (Fig: 2.87).
- At the end of application rub the tape until the warmth is felt, this is necessary to activate the glue.

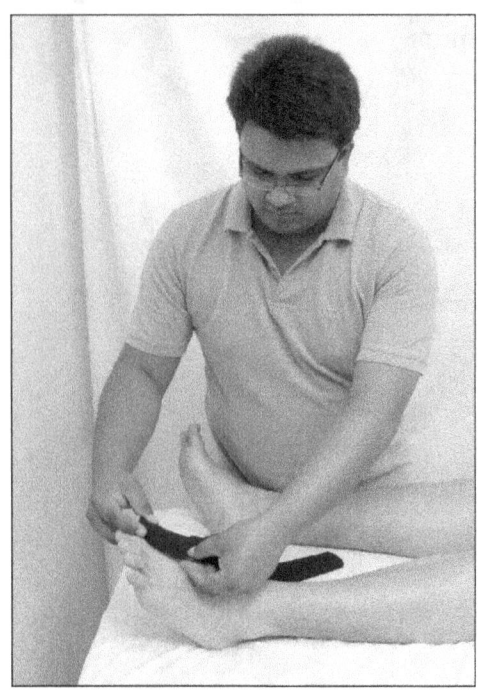

Figure 2.85: Measuring the tape.

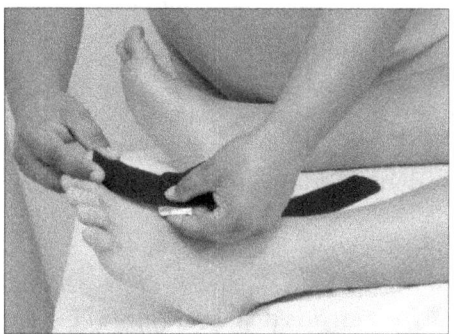

Figure 2.86: Application of base.

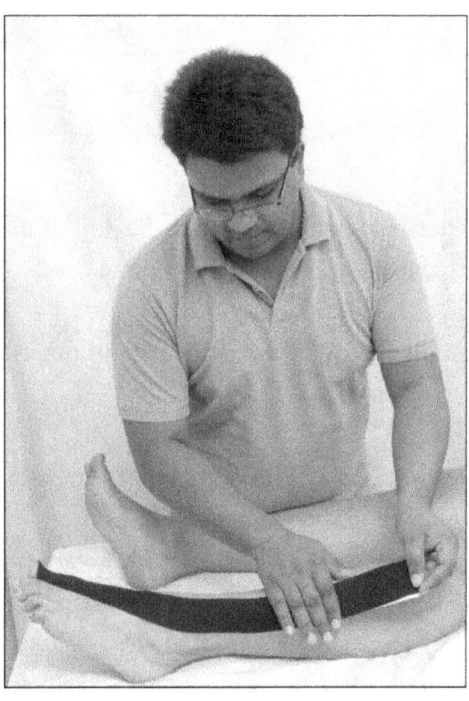

Figure 2.87: Application of tail.

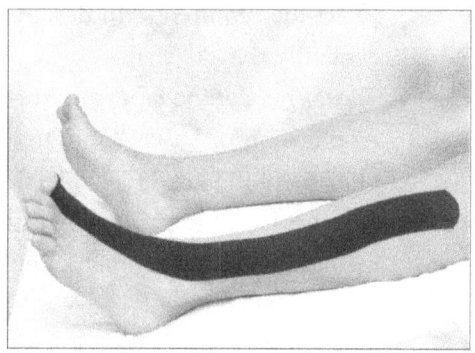

Figure 2.88: Final application.

# Internal Abdominal Oblique

**Technique used**: Muscle tonus up Technique.

**Muscle:** Internal abdominal oblique.

**Origin:**

- Thoraco-lumbar fascia,
- Anterior 2/3 of the iliac crest,
- Lateral 2/3 of the inguinal ligament.

**Insertion:**

- Lower 3 or 4 ribs,
- Linea alba,
- Pubic crest.

**Function:** Flexes and laterally bends the trunk.

**Innervation:** Intercostal nerves T 7-T11, subcostal, iliohypogastric and ilioinguinal nerves.

**Subject's position:** Supine Lying.

**Therapist position:** Standing next to the subject.

**Strip**: I shaped tape is used.

**Procedure:**

- Follow the basic steps for muscle taping.
- Measuring the tape: The subject is asked to flex the knee so as the feet touches the couch, and laterally flex the hip and trunk on the same side of application so as to stretch the muscle. The tape is measured from iliac crest to linea alba at 4th rib position (Fig: 2.89).
- Select the required strip design, for large muscle bulk, use "I" strip and in small muscle generally the "Y" strip.
- The corners of the tapes are rounded off.
- Application of base: Apply the base with no stretch just distal to the iliac crest (Fig: 2.90).
- Application of the tail: When subject's muscle is in stretched position, therapist stabilizes the base with one hand and applies the rest of the tape with paper off or 10% stretch (Fig: 2.91).
- At the end of application rub the tape until the warmth is felt, this is necessary to activate the glue.

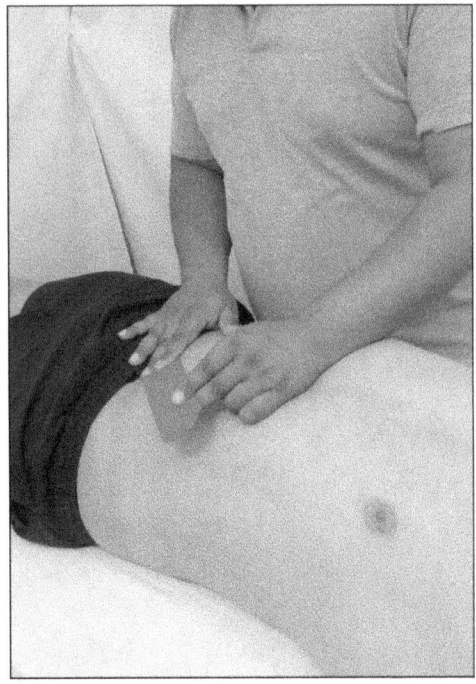

Figure 2.89: Measuring the tape.

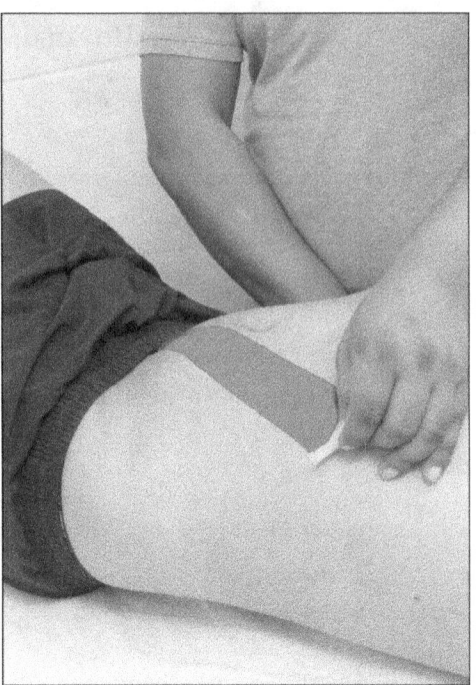

Figure 2.90: Application of base.

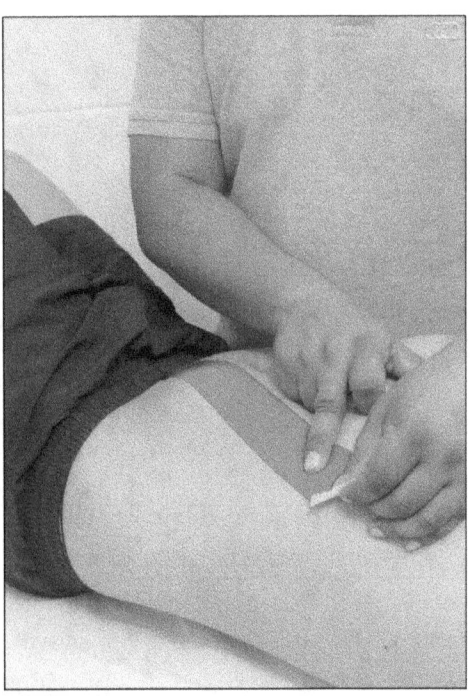

Figure 2.91: Application of tail.

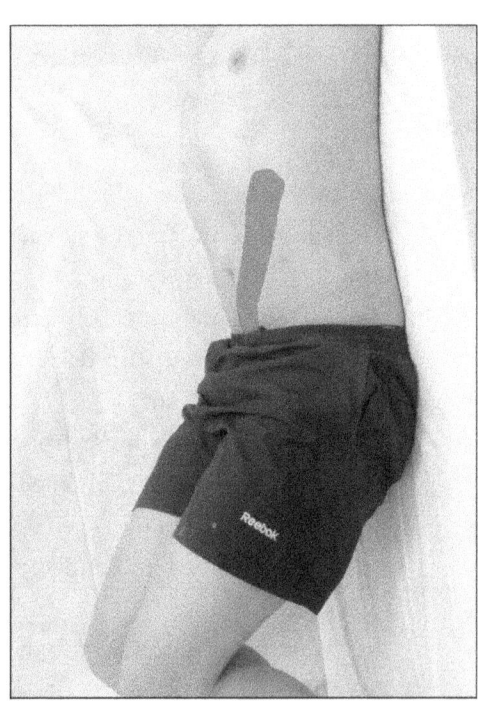

Figure 2.92: Final application.

# External Abdominal Oblique

**Technique used**: Muscle tonus down Technique.

**Muscle**: External Abdominal Oblique[23].

**Origin:**

- Lower 8 Ribs.

**Insertion:**

- Linea alba, pubic crest & tubercle,
- Anterior superior iliac spine ,
- Anterior half of iliac crest.

**Function:**

- Flexes and laterally bends the trunk.

**Innervation:**

- Intercostal nerves T7-T11,
- Subcostal,
- Iliohypogastric and ilioinguinal nerves.

**Subject's position:** Supine Lying.

**Therapist position**: Therapist standing next to the subject.

**Strip:** I shaped tape is used.

**Procedure:**

- Follow the basic steps for muscle taping
- Measuring the tape: The subject is asked to flex the knee so as the feet touches the couch, and laterally flex the hip and trunk to the opposite side of application so as to stretch the muscle. The tape is measured from anterior superior iliac spine to mid clavicular line at 8th rib (Fig: 2.93).
- Select the required strip design, for large muscle bulk, use "I" strip and in small muscle generally the "Y" strip.
- The corners of the tapes are rounded off.
- Application of base: Apply the base with no stretch just distal to the ASIS (Fig: 2.94).
- Application of the tail: When subject's muscle is in stretched position, therapist stabilizes the base with one hand and applies the rest of the tape with paper off or 10% stretch (Fig: 2.95).
- At the end of application rub the tape until the warmth is felt, this is necessary to activate the glue.

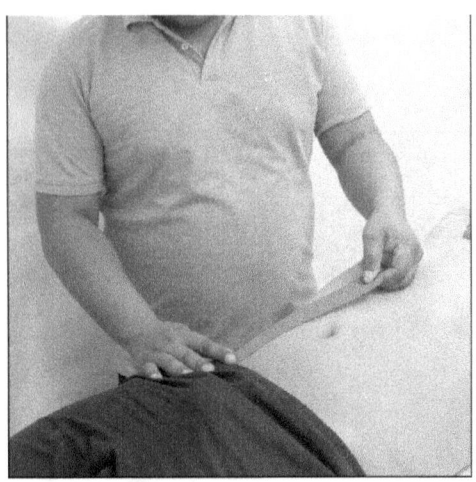

Figure 2.93: Measuring the tape.

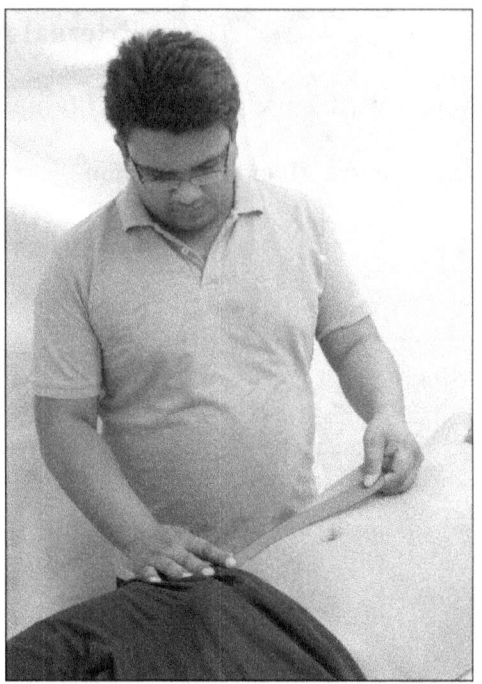

Figure 2.94: Application of base.

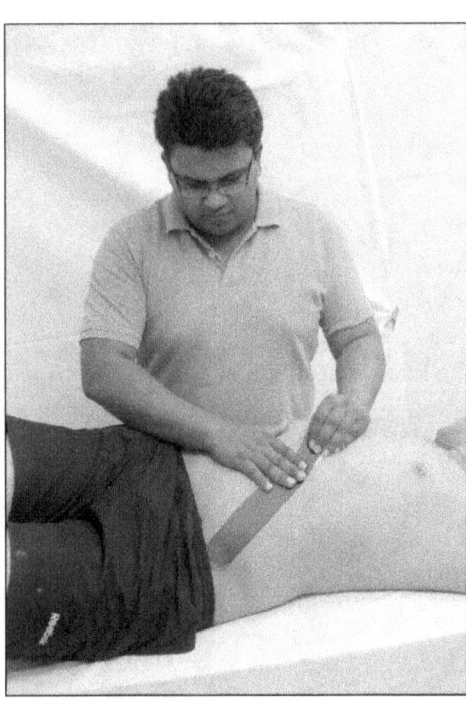

Figure 2.95: Application of tail.

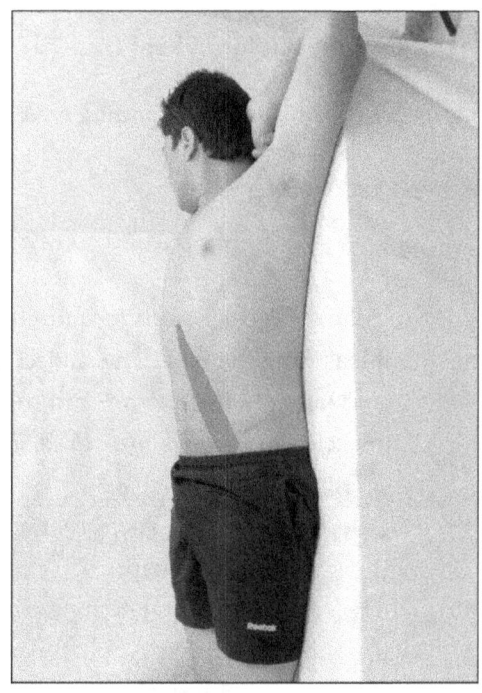

Figure 2.96: Final application.

# Errector Spinae

**Technique used**: Muscle tonus up Technique.

**Muscle:** Errector Spinae. The erector spinae muscle is separated into 3 columns of muscle: Iliocostalis laterally, Longissimus in an intermediate position and Spinalis medially[87].

## Origin:

- Iliac crest and sacrum,
- Transverse and spinous processes of vertebrae,
- Supraspinal ligament.

Iliocostalis
- Lower posterior surface of the sacrum,
- Posterior surface of the ribs.

Longissimus
- Transverse processes of the sacrum, lumbar vertebrae and thoracic vertebrae.

Spinalis
- Transverse processes of the cervical and thoracic vertebrae,
- Posterior neck ligaments of the ligamentum nuchae.

## Insertion:

- Angles of the ribs,
- Transverse and spinous processes of vertebrae,
- Posterior aspect of the skull.

Iliocostalis
- Posterior surface of the ribs,
- Transverse processes of the cervical vertebrae.

Longissimus
- Transverse processes of the cervical and thoracic vertebrae,
- Mastoid process of the skull.

Spinalis
- Spinous processes of the cervical and thoracic vertebrae.

**Innervation:** By dorsal primary rami of spinal nerves C1-S 5.

**Function:** Extends and laterally bends the trunk, neck and head.

Iliocostalis and Longissimus

- Bilateral flexion of the cervical, lumbar and thoracic spine,
- Extension and rotation of the cervical, lumbar and thoracic spine.

Spinalis

- Bilateral flexion and rotation of the cervical spine,
- Extension of the cervical, lumbar and thoracic spine.

**Subject's position:** Subject standing in comfortable position.

**Therapist position:** Therapist standing at the back of the subject.

**Strip:** Y shaped tape is used.

**Procedure:**

- Follow the basic steps for muscle taping.
- Measuring the tape: The subject is asked to do trunk forward flexion, the tape is measured from L5-S1 vertebrae till the T5-T6 level (Fig: 2.97).
- Select the required strip design, for large muscle bulk, use "I" strip and in small muscle generally the "Y" strip.
- The corners of the tapes are rounded off.
- Application of base: Apply the base with no stretch just distal to the L5 (Fig: 2.98).
- Application of the tail: When subject's muscle is in stretched position, therapist stabilizes the base with one hand and applies the rest of the tape with paper off or 10% stretch (Fig: 2.99).
- At the end of application rub the tape until the warmth is felt, this is necessary to activate the glue.

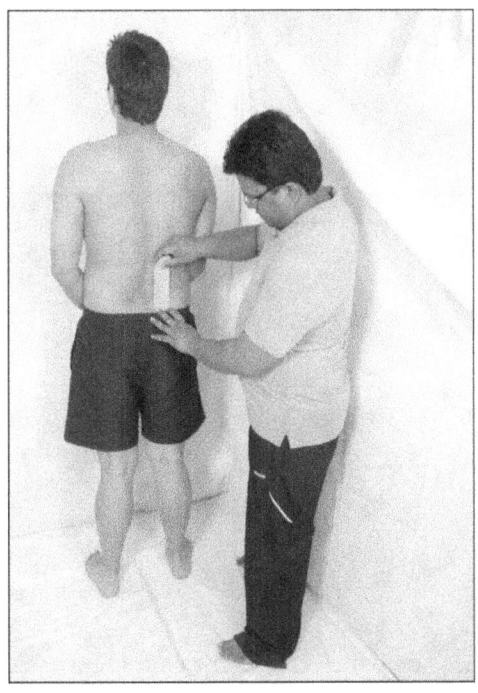

Figure 2.97: Measuring the tape.

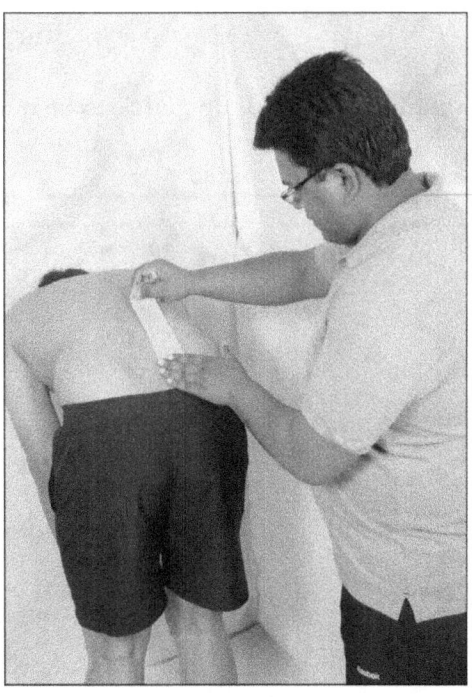

Figure 2.98: Application of base.

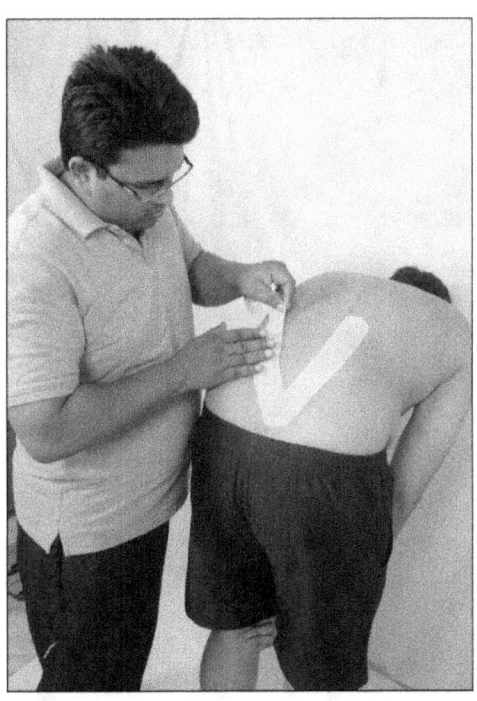

Figure 2.99: Application of tail.

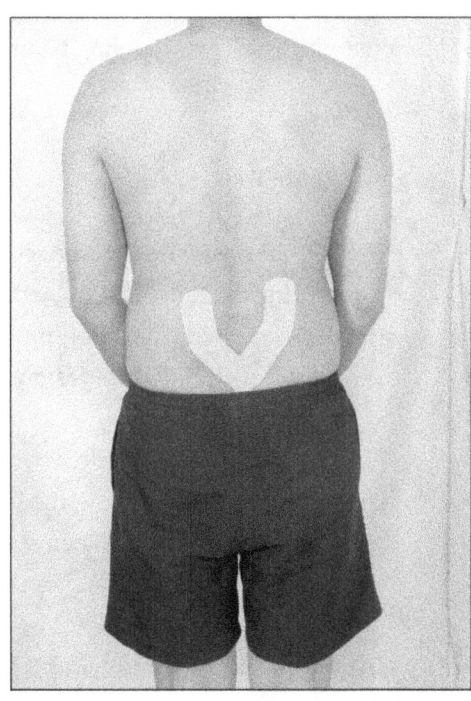

Figure 2.100: Final application.

# Sternocledomastoid

**Technique Used**: Tonus up muscle technique

**Muscle**: Sternocledomastoid.

**Origin**:

- Sternal head: anterior surface of the manubrium;
- Clavicularhead: medial 1/3rd of the clavicle.

**Insertion**:

- Mastoid process ,
- Lateral 1/2 of the superior nuchal line.

**Function**:

- Draws the mastoid process down toward the same side which causes the chin to turn up toward the opposite side,
- Acting together, the muscles of the two sides flex the neck.

**Innervations**: Spinal Accessory Nerve (XI), with sensory supply from C2 & C3.

**Subject Position**: Subject sitting in relaxed comfortable position.

**Therapist Position**: Therapist standing behind the subject.

**Strip**: I strip is used.

**Procedure**:

- Follow the basic steps for muscle taping.
- Measuring the tape: The subject is asked to side flex and rotate neck to same side and the tape is measured from sternum manubrium to the mastoid process. (Fig: 2.101)
- Select the required strip design, for large muscle bulk, use "I" strip and in small muscle generally the "Y" strip.
- The corners of the tapes are rounded off.
- Application of base: Apply the base with no stretch just on distal to the manubrium .
- Application of the tail: When subject's muscle is in stretched position, therapist stabilizes the base with one hand and applies the rest of the tape with paper off or 10% stretch (Fig: 2.102).
- At the end of application rub the tape until the warmth is felt, this is necessary to activate the glue.

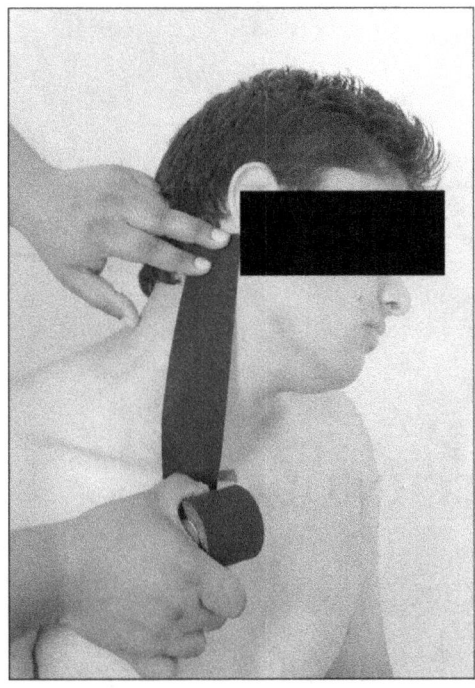

Figure 2.101: Measuring the tape.

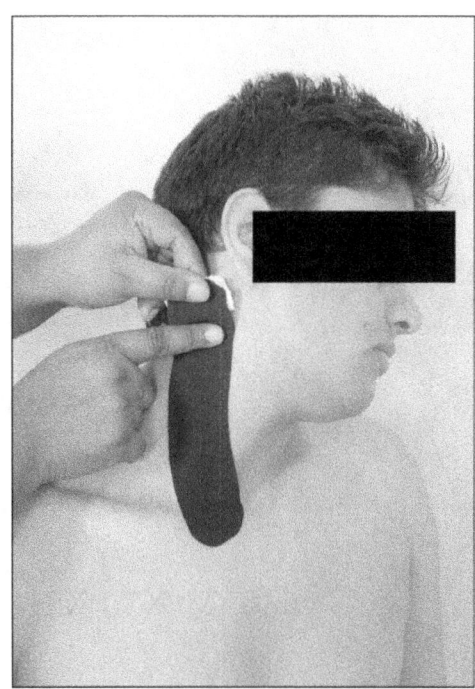

Figure 2.102: Application of tail.

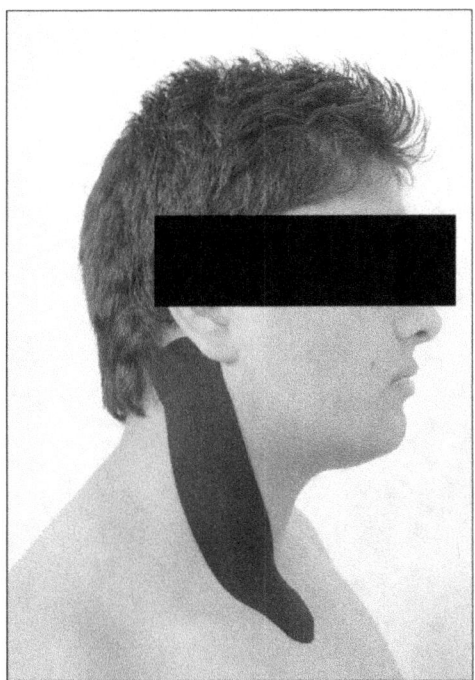

Figure 2.103: Final application.

# CHAPTER 3

# LIGAMENT TAPING TECHNIQUE

(LIGAMENT TECHNIQUE & SPACE TECHNIQUE)

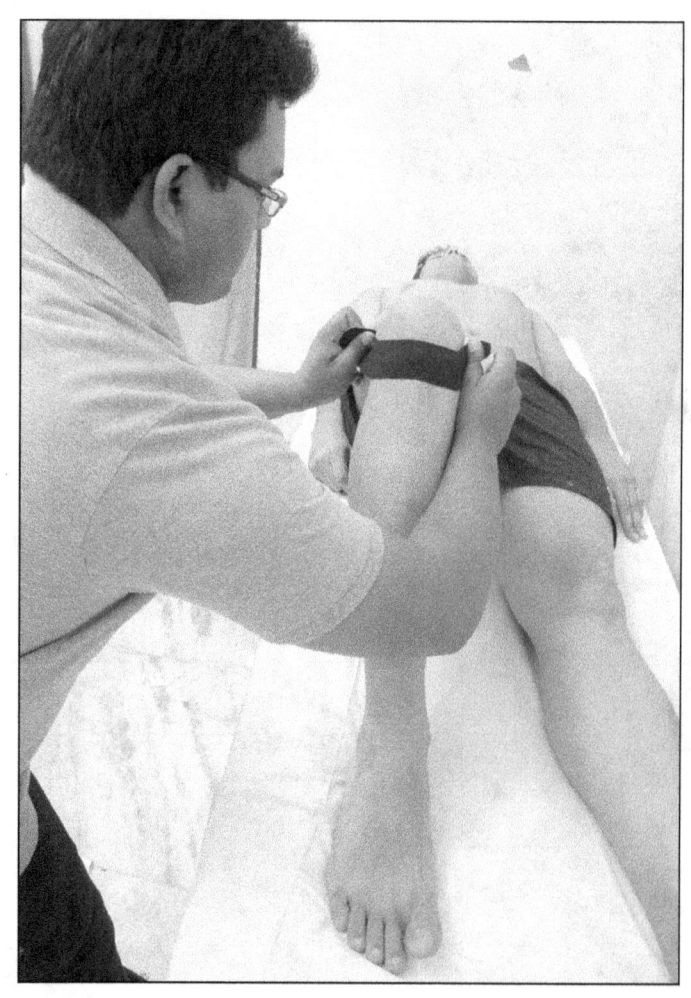

# Ligament Taping Technique (Ligament Application & Space Technique)

Ligament taping techniques are used to provide static as well as dynamic stability to ligamentous structures and the joints. The ligaments are the fibrous tissues that connect one bone to other bone. "Ligament" is most commonly referred to a band of tough, fibrous dense regular connective tissue comprising attenuated collagenous fibres. Ligaments are visco-elastic; they gradually lengthen under tension, and return to their original shape when the tension is removed. However, they cannot retain their original shape when stretched past a certain point or for a prolonged period of time. This is one reason why dislocated joints must be reduced as quickly as possible: if the ligaments lengthen too much, then the joint will be loose its stability, becoming prone to future dislocations[20].

The kinesiological taping is use to provide additional dynamic stability to the ligaments. Where conventional taping methods provide static stability to the ligament structure, the kinesiological taping provides dynamic stability.[20,41]

The tearing of backing paper for this technique differs from that of muscle technique, as in this we tear the paper from centre and fold it to both sides, making only the middle part of the tape to be exposed, the tape is then stretched evenly from both sides with 50%-75% stretch. The centre is applied with stretch while the joint is in neutral position, and then the subject is instructed to move the joint while the therapist applies the rest of the tape with the movement except the end of the tape which are applied without stretch[41].

## Action of the tape

As both ends of the tape are the bases which are applied unstretched while centre of the tape is stretched, the middle will recoil making the bases to move towards the centre hence stabilizing the ligaments. As the tape is applied when the joint was in motion it will not restrict the movement of the joint. The collateral ligaments are best to treat with this method.

General steps for ligament techniques:

- Evaluation: This is the prerequisite of every therapy, the subject must be evaluated and the structure at fault is diagnosed and selection of taping technique is done.
- Part of the subject should be completely clean from dirt and oil and in case of excessive body hair, it should be shaved off.
- Measuring the tape: The subject is asked to move the joint and the tape is measured 2cm above and below the attachment of the ligament across the joint.
- Select the required strip design: For large muscle belly the "Y" strip is used and in flat muscle generally the "I" strip is used.
- The corners of the tapes are rounded off.
- Application of tape: The backing paper of the tape strip is torn from the middle, the tape is stretched to 50% to 75% from the middle while the ends of the tape are kept unstretched, and the tape is applied while the joint is in motion. The ends are applied without stretch.

- At the end of application rub the tape until the warmth is felt, this is necessary to activate the glue.

# Sternoclavicular Ligament

**Technique used**: Ligament Technique.

**Structure**: Sternoclavicular Ligament.

**Attachments:** The sternoclavicular ligament has two parts: anterior and posterior. It is a very strong ligament.

- Anterior sternoclavicular ligament is attached above to the upper and front part of the sternal end of the clavicle, and, below to the front of the upper part of the manubrium sterni.
- The posterior sternoclavicular ligament is attached above to the upper and backpart of the sternal end of the clavicle, and, passing obliquely downward and medially and, is fixed below to the back of the upper part of the manubrium sterni.

**Function**:

- It reinforces the capsule of the sternoclavicular joint.
- Stabilizes the sternoclavicular joint.

**Subject position**: Subject sitting in relaxed comfortable position.

**Therapist position**: Therapist standing in front of the subject.

**Strip**: I-strip is used.

**Procedure:**

- Follow the basic steps for ligament taping.
- Measuring the tape: The tape strip size depends on the physique of the subject. The strip should be 2cm more in length than the application area.
- Select the required strip design, generally "I" strips are used.
- The corners of the tapes are rounded off.
- Application of tape: The backing paper is torn off from center, the tape is stretched to 75-100% of its length, the center of tape is applied and both the ends are attached without any stretch. The application is repeated with 2 strips if needed. First strip is always parallel to the ligament attachment (Fig: 3.1).
- At the end of application rub the tape until the warmth is felt, this is necessary to activate the glue.

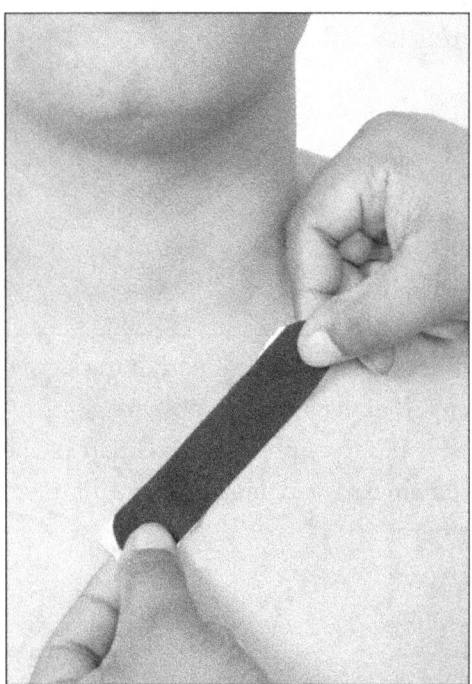

Figure 3.1: Application of strip.

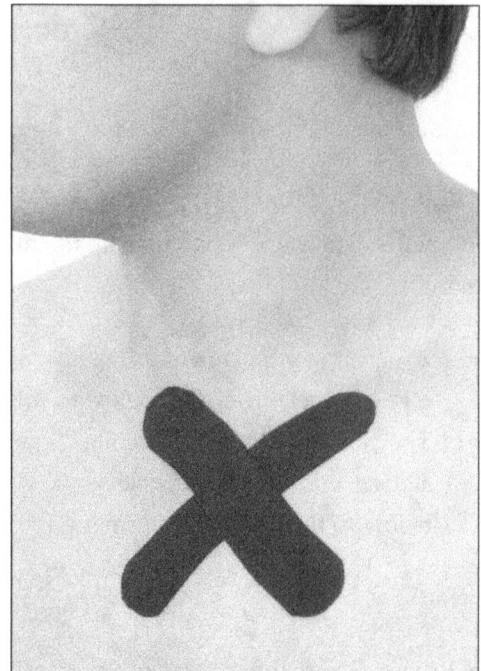

Figure 3.2: Final application.

# Acromioclavicular Ligament

**Technique used**: Ligament Technique.

**Structure**: Acromioclavicular Ligament.

**Attachments:** The Acromioclavicular ligament has two parts: Superior and inferior.

- Superior Acromioclavicular Ligament-This ligament is a quadrilateral band, covering the superior part of the articulation, and extending between the upper part of the lateral end of the clavicle and the adjoining part of the upper surface of the acromion.
- Inferior Acromioclavicular Ligament- This ligament is somewhat thinner than the preceding. It covers the under part of the articulation, and is attached to the adjoining surfaces of the two bones.

**Function**:

- Acromioclavicular ligaments prevent distal clavicular rotation.
- Acromioclavicular ligaments prevent anterior and posterior translation of clavicle.

**Subject position**: Subject sitting in relaxed comfortable position.

**Therapist position**: Therapist standing behind the subject.

**Strip**: I-strip is used.

**Procedure:**

- Follow the basic steps for ligament taping.
- Measuring the tape:  The tape strip size depends on the physique of the subject. The strip should be 2cm more in length than the application area.
- Select the required strip design, generally "I" strips are used.
- The corners of the tapes are rounded off.
- Application of tape: The backing paper is torn off from center, the tape is stretched to 75-100% of its length, the center of tape is applied and both the ends are attached without any stretch. The application is repeated with 2 strips if needed. First strip is always parallel to the ligament attachment (Fig: 3.3).
- At the end of application rub the tape until the warmth is felt, this is necessary to activate the glue.

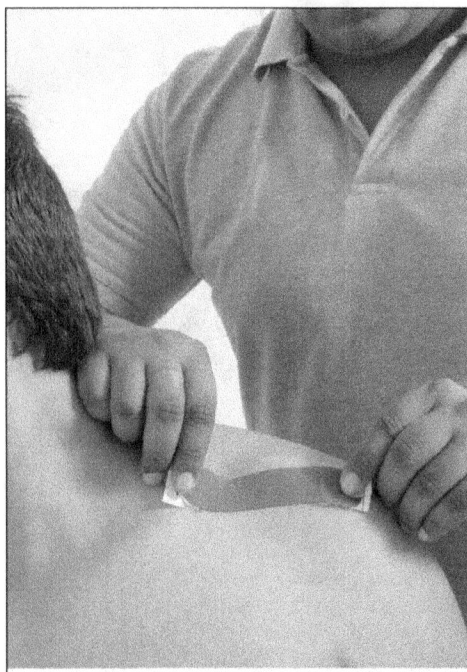

Figure 3.3: Application of strip.

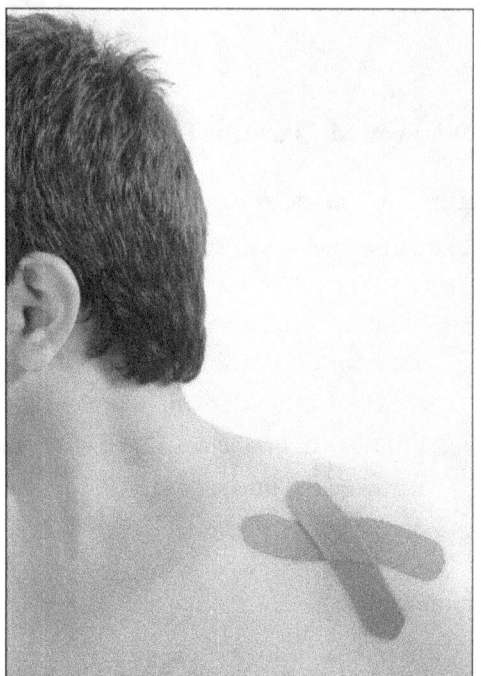

Figure 3.4: Final application.

## Medial Collateral Ligament of Elbow (Ulnar Collateral Ligament)

**Technique used**: Ligament Technique.

**Structure**: Medial Collateral Ligament.

**Attachments:** It is a strong ligament of elbow spanning through the medial side of the elbow joint that connects the medial epicondyle of the humerus with the ulna.

**Function**:

- It reinforces the medial side of the elbow articular capsule.
- It is a primary medial stabilizer of the flexed elbow joint.
- In full extension MCL provides about 30 % of stability to elbow joint.

**Subject position**: Subject sitting in relaxed comfortable position.

**Therapist position**: Therapist standing in front of the subject.

**Strip**: I-strip is used.

**Procedure:**

- Follow the basic steps for ligament taping.
- Measuring the tape: The tape strip size depends on the physique of the subject. The strip should be 2cm more in length than the application area.
- Select the required strip design, generally "I" strips are used.
- The corners of the tapes are rounded off.
- Application of tape: The backing paper is torn off from center, the tape is stretched to 75-100% of its length, the center of tape is applied while the subject is moving the elbow into flexion, and both the ends are attached without any stretch. The application is repeated with 2 strips if needed. First strip is always parallel to the ligament attachment (Fig: 3.5, fig 3.6).
- At the end of application rub the tape until the warmth is felt, this is necessary to activate the glue.

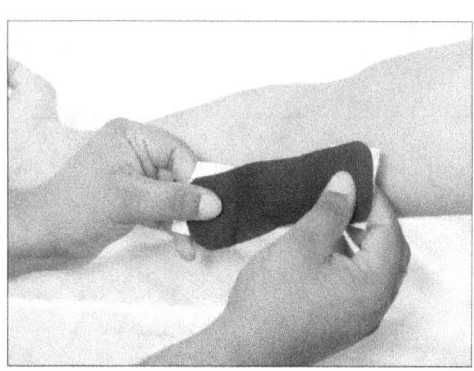

Figure 3.5: Application of strip.

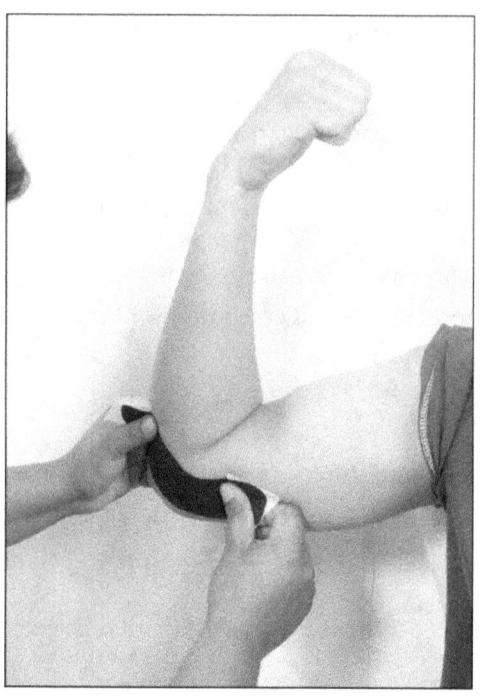

Figure 3.6: Application of strip during flexion.

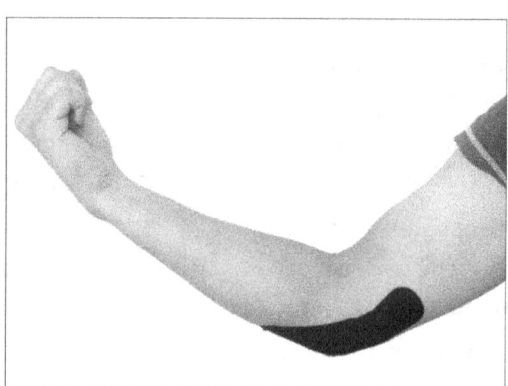

Figure 3.7: Final application.

## Lateral Collateral Ligament of Elbow (Radial Collateral Ligament)

**Technique used**: Ligament Technique.

**Structure**: Lateral Collateral Ligament[6].

**Attachments** This ligament spans to the lateral side of the elbow joint. It connects the lateral epicondyle of the humerus with the radius and the annular ligament.

**Function**:

- It reinforces the lateral side of the elbow articular capsule,
- Stabilizer against posterolateral rotational instability,
- Taut throughout entire range of motion of the elbow.

**Subject position**: Subject sitting in relaxed comfortable position with elbow extended.

**Therapist position**: Therapist standing behind the subject.

**Strip**: I-strip is used.

**Procedure**:

- Follow the basic steps for ligament taping.
- Measuring the tape: The tape strip size depends on the physique of the subject. The strip should be 2cm more in length than the application area.
- Select the required strip design, generally "I" strips are used.
- The corners of the tapes are rounded off.
- Application of tape: The backing paper is torn off from center, the tape is stretched to 75-100% of its length, the center of tape is applied while the subject is moving the elbow into flexion, and both the ends are attached without any stretch. The application is repeated with 2 strips if needed. First strip is always parallel to the ligament attachment (Fig: 3.8).
- At the end of application rub the tape until the warmth is felt, this is necessary to activate the glue.

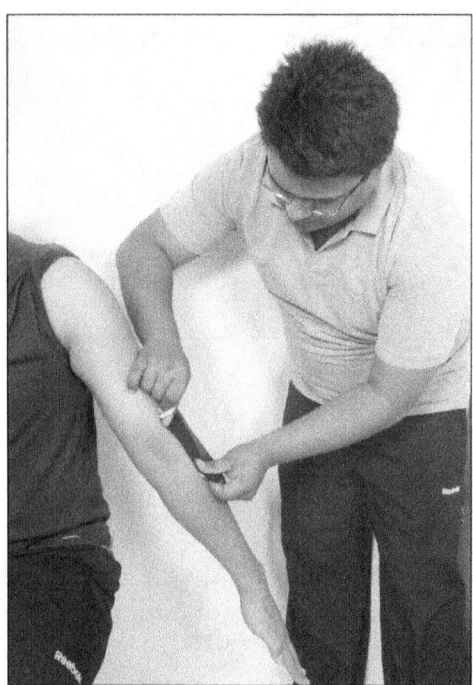

Figure 3.8: Application of centre of strip.

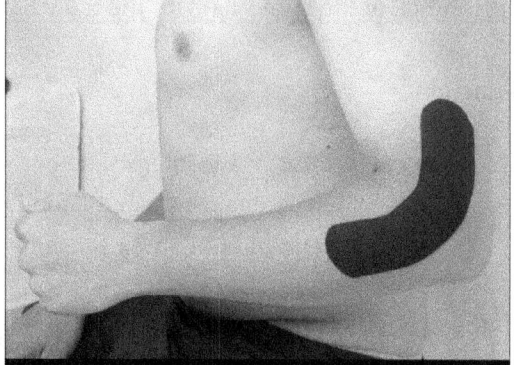

Figure 3.9: Final application.

# Medial Collateral Ligament of Knee (Tibial Collateral Ligament)

**Technique used**: Ligament Technique.

**Structure**: Medial Collateral Ligament.

**Attachments** This ligament connects the medial epicondyle of the femur with the medial surface of the medial condyle of the tibia. It is attached to the medial meniscus which has clinical relevance.

**Function**:

- It provides primary restraint to valgus stress at knee.
- Stabilizes the hinge-like motion of the knee and prevents knee abduction.
- The tibial collateral ligament reinforces the medial surface of the articular capsule of the knee[65].

**Subject position**: Subject supine lying in relaxed comfortable position.

**Therapist position**: Therapist standing at side of the subject.

**Strip**: I-strip is used.

**Procedure:**

- Follow the basic steps for ligament taping.
- Measuring the tape: The tape strip size depends on the physique of the subject. The strip should be 2cm more in length than the application area.
- Select the required strip design, generally "I" strips are used.
- The corners of the tapes are rounded off.
- Application of tape: The backing paper is torn off from center, the tape is stretched to 75-100% of its length, the center of tape is applied while the subject is moving the knee into flexion, and both the ends are attached without any stretch. The application is repeated with 2 strips if needed. First strip is always parallel to the ligament attachment (Fig: 3.10, fig 3.11).
- At the end of application rub the tape until the warmth is felt, this is necessary to activate the glue.

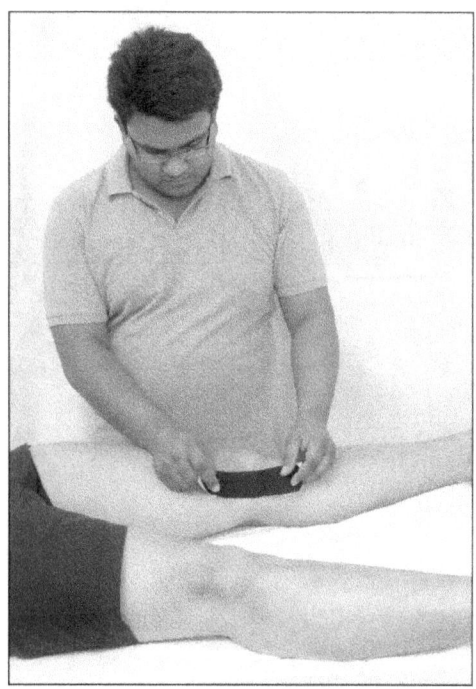

Figure 3.10: Application of strip.

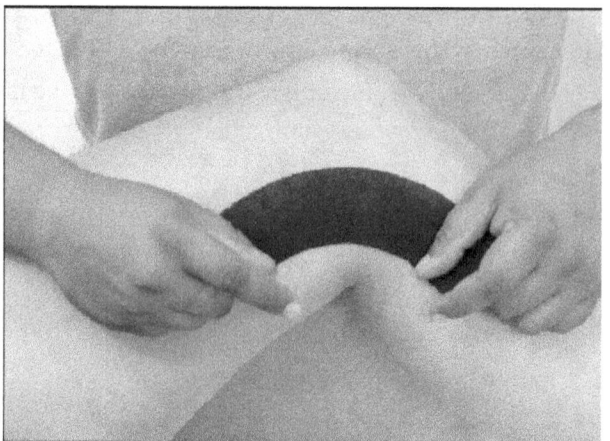

Figure 3.11: Application of strip during flexion.

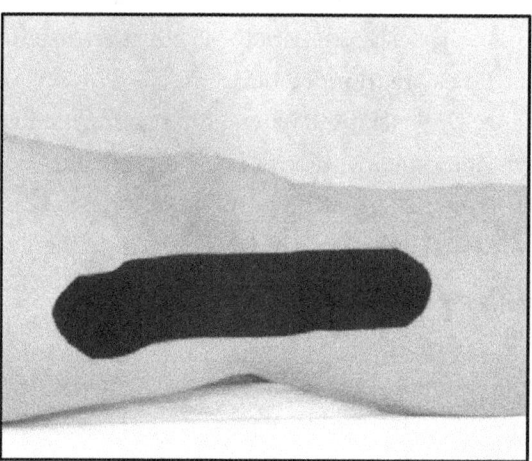

Figure 3.12: Final application.

# Lateral Collateral Ligament of Knee (Fibular Collateral Ligament)

**Technique used**: Ligament Technique.

**Structure**: Lateral Collateral Ligament.

**Attachments** It connects the lateral epicondyle of the femur with the head of the fibula.

- It attaches superiorly to the lateral femoral epicondyle just above the groove for the popliteus tendon.
- Inferiorly, it is attached to a depression on the lateral surface of the fibular head.

**Function**:

- Primary restraint to varus stress of the knee.
- Resists tibial external rotation.

**Subject position**: Subject supine lying in relaxed comfortable position[65].

**Therapist position**: Therapist standing at the side of the subject.

**Strip**: I-strip is used.

**Procedure**:

- Follow the basic steps for ligament taping.
- Measuring the tape: The tape strip size depends on the physique of the subject. The strip should be 2cm more in length than the application area.
- Select the required strip design, generally "I" strips are used.
- The corners of the tapes are rounded off.
- Application of tape: The backing paper is torn off from center, the tape is stretched to 75-100% of its length, the center of tape is applied while the subject is moving the knee into flexion, and both the ends are attached without any stretch. The application is repeated with 2 strips if needed. First strip is always parallel to the ligament attachment (Fig: 3.13, fig 3.14).
- At the end of application rub the tape until the warmth is felt, this is necessary to activate the glue.

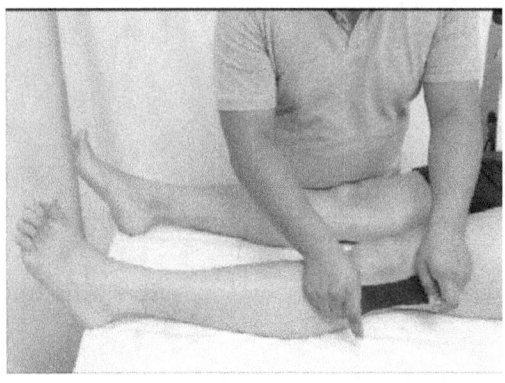

Figure 3.13: Application of strip.

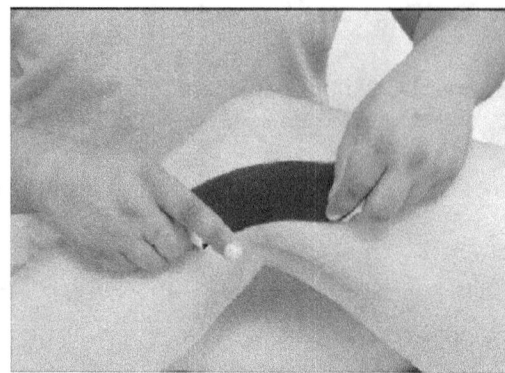

Figure 3.14: Application of strip during flexion.

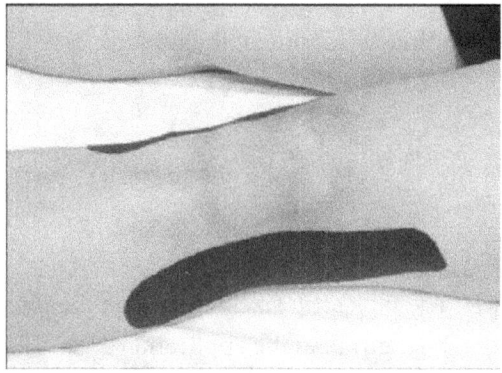

Figure 3.15: Final application.

## Anterior Cruciate Ligament of Knee

**Technique used**: Ligament Technique.

**Structure**: Anterior Cruciate Ligament.

**Attachments** It connects the lateral epicondyle of the femur with the head of the fibula.

- It attaches superiorly to the lateral wall of the intercondylar notch at its posterior aspect,
- Inferiorly, it is attached to an Oval shaped area, anterior aspect of the tibial plateau between the tibial eminences.

**Function**:

- Prevents hyperextension and excessive internal rotation.
- The anterior cruciate ligament limits the anterior movement of the tibia relative to the femur in all positions of joint movement[61].

**Subject position**: Subject supine lying in relaxed comfortable position.

**Therapist position**: Therapist standing at the foot end of the subject.

**Strip**: I-strip is used.

**Procedure:**

- Follow the basic steps for ligament taping.
- Measuring the tape: The tape strip size depends on the physique of the subject. The strip should be 2cm more in length than the application area.
- Select the required strip design, generally "I" strips are used.
- The corners of the tapes are rounded off.
- Application of tape: The backing paper is torn off from center, the tape is stretched to 75-100% of its length, the center of tape is applied anteriorly just below the inferior pole of patella while the subject is moving the knee into flexion, and both the ends are attached without any stretch. The application is repeated with 2 strips if needed. First strip is always parallel to the ligament attachment (Fig: 3.16).
- At the end of application rub the tape until the warmth is felt, this is necessary to activate the glue.

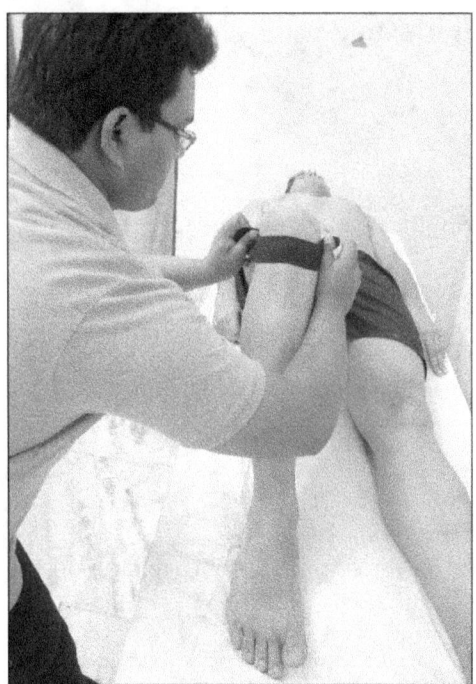

Figure 3.16: Application of strip.

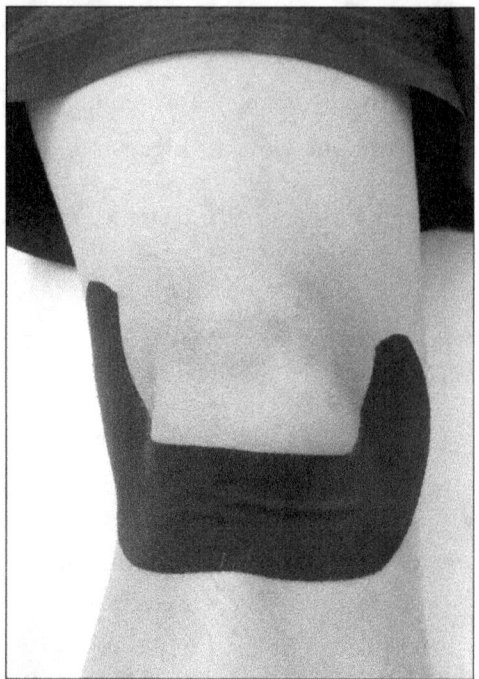

Figure 3.17: Final application.

# Lateral Collateral Ligament of Ankle

**Technique used**: Ligament Technique.

**Structure**:Lateral Collateral Ligament.

**Attachments:**

- Anterior Talofibular Ligament -A ligament that connects the lateral malleolus of the fibula with the anterolateral surface of the talus.
- Posterior Talofibular Ligament- A ligament that connects the lateral malleolus of the fibula with the posterolateral surface of the talus.
- Calcaneofibular Ligament-A ligament that connects the lateral malleolus of the fibula with the calcaneus.

**Function:**

- Lateral collateral ligament of ankle reinforces the ankle joint laterally[1,85].

**Subject position**: Subject supine lying with foot resting on the couch.

**Therapist position**: Therapist standing at the side of the subject.

**Strip**: I-strip is used.

**Procedure:**

- Follow the basic steps for ligament taping.
- Measuring the tape:  The tape strip size depends on the physique of the subject. The strip should be 2cm more in length than the application area.
- Select the required strip design, generally "I" strips are used.
- The corners of the tapes are rounded off.
- Application of tape: The backing paper is torn off from center, the tape is stretched to 75-100% of its length, the center of tape is applied to the middle of each ligament length and both the ends are attached without any stretch. The application is repeated with 2 strips if needed. First strip is always parallel to the ligament attachment (Fig: 3.18, Fig: 3.19).
- At the end of application rub the tape until the warmth is felt, this is necessary to activate the glue.

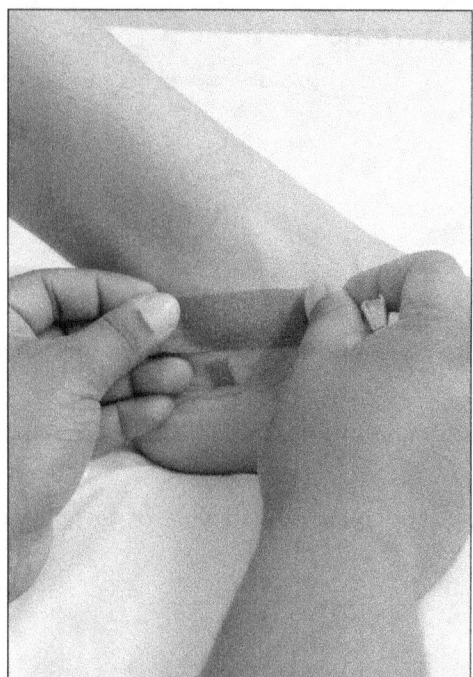

Figure 3.18: Application of strip.

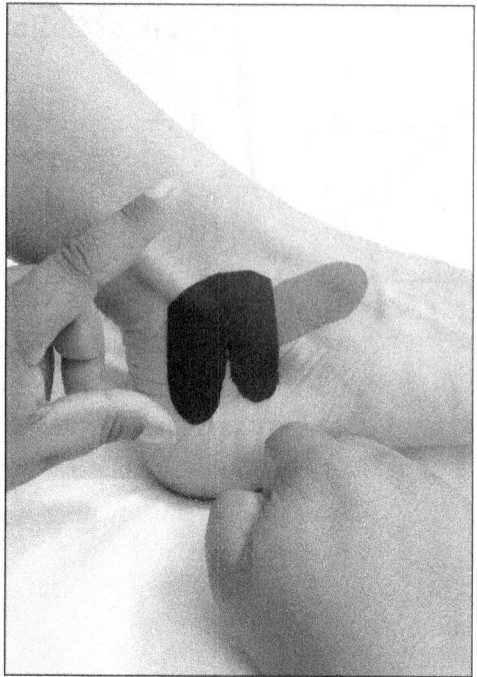

Figure 3.19: Final application.

# Medial Collateral Ligament of Ankle

**Technique used**: Ligament Technique.

**Structure**: Medial Collateral Ligament.

**Attachments**It has four parts (from anterior to posterior):

- Anterior Tibiotalar Ligament- It is a part of the deltoid ligament connecting the medial malleolus of the tibia with the talus.
- Tibionavicular Ligament-It is a part of the deltoid ligament connecting the medial malleolus of the tibia with the navicular.
- Tibiocalcaneal Ligament- It is a part of the deltoid ligament connecting the medial malleolus of the tibia with the sustentaculum tali.
- Posterior Tibiotalar Ligament- It is a part of the deltoid ligament connecting the medial malleolus of the tibia with the talus posteriorly.

**Function**:

- The deltoid ligament reinforces the ankle joint medially[85].

**Subject position**: Subject supine lying with foot resting on the bed.

**Therapist position**: Therapist standing at the side of the subject.

**Strip**: I-strip is used.

**Procedure**:

- Follow the basic steps for ligament taping.
- Measuring the tape:  The tape strip size depends on the physique of the subject. The strip should be 2cm more in length than the application area.
- Select the required strip design, generally "I" strips are used.
- The corners of the tapes are rounded off.
- Application of tape: The backing paper is torn off from center, the tape is stretched to 75-100% of its length, the center of tape is applied to the middle of each ligament length and both the ends are attached without any stretch. The application is repeated with 2 strips if needed. First strip is always parallel to the ligament attachment (Fig: 3.20, Fig: 3.21).
- At the end of application rub the tape until the warmth is felt, this is necessary to activate the glue.

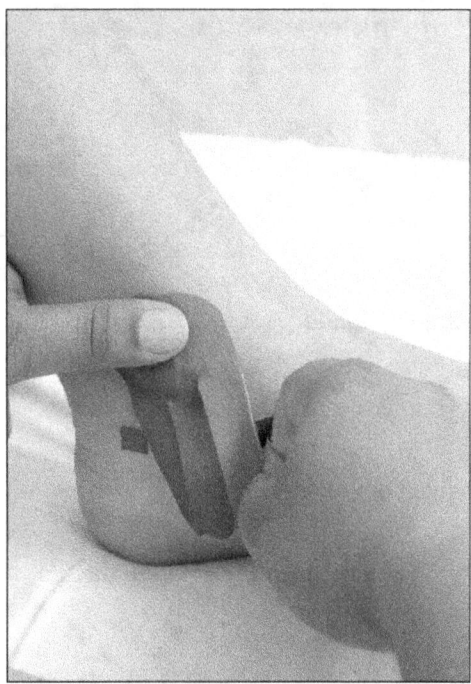

Figure 3.20: Application of strip.

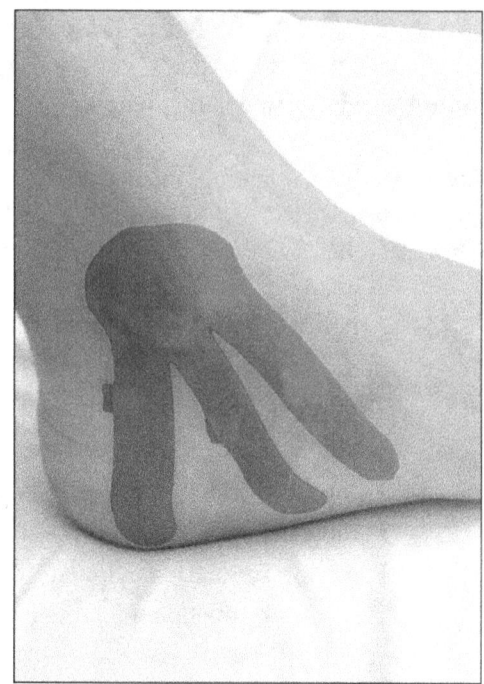

Figure 3.21:  Final application.

# Space Tape Techniques

Space taping technique is a pain relieving technique which is used on trigger points of the body. Trigger points are hyper irritable spots in skeletal muscle that are associated with palpable nodules in taut bands of muscle fibres. Trigger points form only in muscles. They form as a local contraction in a small number of muscle fibres or in a larger muscle or muscle bundle[10]. These in turn can pull on tendons and ligaments associated with the muscle and can cause pain deep within a joint where there are no muscles. When muscle fibres contract, they lead to accumulation of fatigue toxins such as lactic acid. The tightened muscle fibres constrict capillaries and prevent them from carrying off the fatigue toxins to the body's recycling system (liver and kidneys). The build-up of these toxins in a muscle bundle makes muscle feels like a tight muscle—a slippery elongate bundle. When trigger points are present in muscles there is often pain and weakness in the associated structures. These pain patterns in muscles follow specific nerve pathways [10,53].

The kinesiological taping is used as a space tape to provide suction cum skin lifting effect just above the trigger points; this activates or stimulates the receptors of skin as well as increase the space below the skin which in turn leads to increase in blood flow which washes away the lactic acid and hence decreasing pain[22].

### Action of the tape

As both the sides are the base and they are unstretched while the centre tape is stretch, the middle of the tape will recoil making the base to contract towards the centre.

General steps for Space techniques:

- Evaluation: This is the prerequisite of every therapy, the subject must be evaluated and the structure at fault is diagnosed and selection of taping technique is done.
- Part of the subject should be completely clean from dirt and oil and in case of excessive body hair, it should be shaved off.
- Measuring the tape: The subject is asked to keep the joint in neutral and the tape is measured from 2cm above to 2 cm below the area of pain or application.
- Select the required strip design, generally the "I" strip is used in space technique, cut 4 strips of same size.
- The corners of the tapes are rounded off.
- Application of tape: The backing paper of the tape strip is torn from the middle, and the application is just like ligament technique with center of tape on pain point while the subject's muscle is in stretched position.
- Apply all the four strips in a plus (+) pattern.
- At the end of application rub the tape until the warmth is felt, this is necessary to activate the glue.

## Brachioradialis (Trigger Point)

**Technique used**: Ligament Technique (Space Technique).

**Structure**: Trigger point brachioradialis[63].

**Indication:**

- Elbow pain.
- Pain in thumb (dorsum).
- Tennis elbow (lateral epicondylitis).
- Weakness in grip.
- Repetitive strain injury.

**Referred pain pattern:** Lateral epicondyle area 3-4cm patch with vague arm pain (radius border), localizing into strong pain in dorsum of thumb.

**Subject position**: Subject sitting in relaxed comfortable position.

**Therapist position**: Therapist standing at the side of the subject.

**Strip**: I-strip is used.

**Procedure:**

- Evaluation: This is the prerequisite of every therapy, the subject must be evaluated and the structure at fault is diagnosed and selection of taping technique is done.
- Part of the subject should be completely clean from dirt and oil and in case of excessive body hair, it should be shaved off.
- Measuring the tape: The subject is asked to keep the joint in neutral and the tape is measured 2cm above and below the area of pain or application.
- Select the required strip design, generally the "I" strip is used in space technique, cut 4 strips of same size.
- The corners of the tapes are rounded off.
- Application of tape: The backing paper of the tape strip is torn from the middle, and the application is just like ligament technique with center of tape is on the pain point while the subject's muscle is in stretched position (Fig: 3.22, Fig: 3.23).
- Apply all the four strips in a plus (+) pattern (Fig: 3.24).
- At the end of application rub the tape until the warmth is felt, this is necessary to activate the glue.

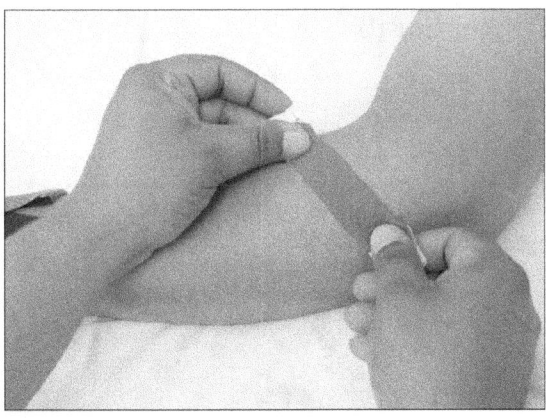

Figure 3.22: Application of strip 1.

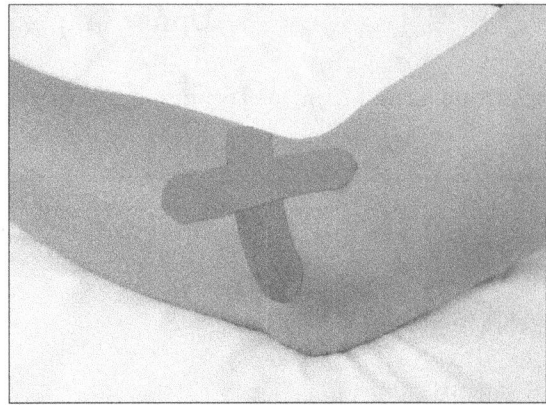

Figure 3.23: Application of strip 2

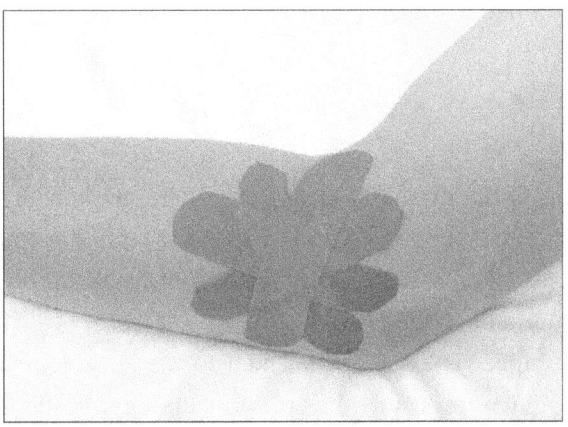

Figure 3.24: Final application.

# Upper Trapezius (Trigger Point)

**Technique used**: Ligament Technique (Space Technique).

**Structure**: Trigger point upper trapezius[64,77].

**Indication:**

- Chronic tension.
- Neck pain.

**Referred pain pattern:** Pain and tenderness, posterior and lateral aspect of upper neck, temporal region and angle of jaw.

**Subject position**: Subject sitting in relaxed comfortable position.

**Therapist position**: Therapist standing at the side of the subject.

**Strip**: I-strip is used.

**Procedure:**

- Evaluation: This is the prerequisite of every therapy, the subject must be evaluated and the structure at fault is diagnosed and selection of taping technique is done.
- Part of the subject should be completely clean from dirt and oil and in case of excessive body hair, it should be shaved off.
- Measuring the tape: The subject is asked to keep the joint in neutral and the tape is measured 2cm above and below the area of pain or application.
- Select the required strip design, generally the "I" strip is used in space technique, cut 4 strips of same size.
- The corners of the tapes are rounded off.
- Application of tape: The backing paper of the tape strip is torn from the middle, and the application is just like ligament technique with center of tape is on the pain point while the subject's muscle is in stretched position (Fig: 3.25, Fig: 3.26).
- Apply all the four strips in a plus (+) pattern (Fig: 3.27).
- At the end of application rub the tape until the warmth is felt, this is necessary to activate the glue.

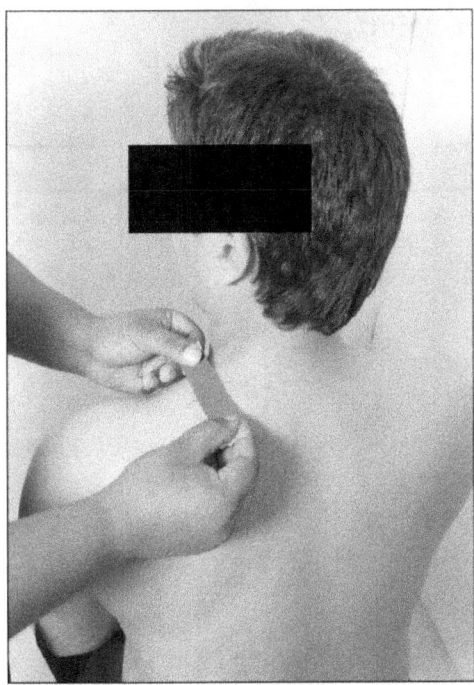

Figure 3.25: Application of strip 1.

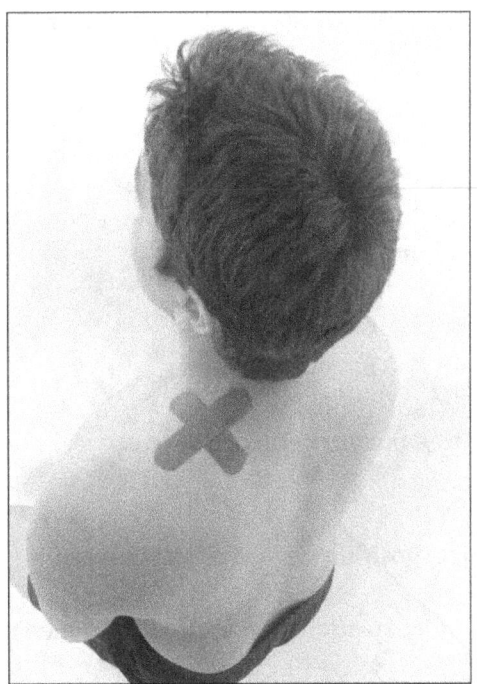

Figure 3.26: Application of strip 2.

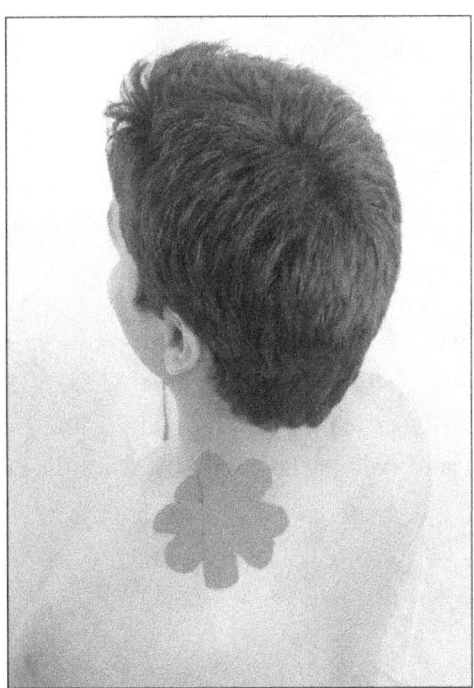

Figure 3.27: Final application of strips.

# Lower Trapezius (Trigger Point)

**Technique used**: Ligament Technique (Space Technique).

**Structure**: Trigger point lower trapezius[64,77].

**Indication:**

- Chronic tension.
- Backache.

**Referred pain pattern:** Posterior cervical spine, mastoid area, area above spine of scapula, upper backache.

**Subject position**: Subject sitting in relaxed comfortable position.

**Therapist position**: Therapist standing behind the subject.

**Strip**: I-strip is used.

**Procedure:**

- Evaluation: This is the prerequisite of every therapy, the subject must be evaluated and the structure at fault is diagnosed and selection of taping technique is done.
- Part of the subject should be completely clean from dirt and oil and in case of excessive body hair, it should be shaved off.
- Measuring the tape: The subject is asked to keep the joint in neutral and the tape is measured 2cm above and below the area of pain or application.
- Select the required strip design, generally the "I" strip is used in space technique, cut 4 strips of same size.
- The corners of the tapes are rounded off.
- Application of tape: The backing paper of the tape strip is torn from the middle, and the application is just like ligament technique with center of tape is on the pain point while the subject's muscle is in stretched position (Fig: 3.28, Fig: 3.29).
- Apply all the four strips in a plus (+) pattern (Fig: 3.30).
- At the end of application rub the tape until the warmth is felt, this is necessary to activate the glue.

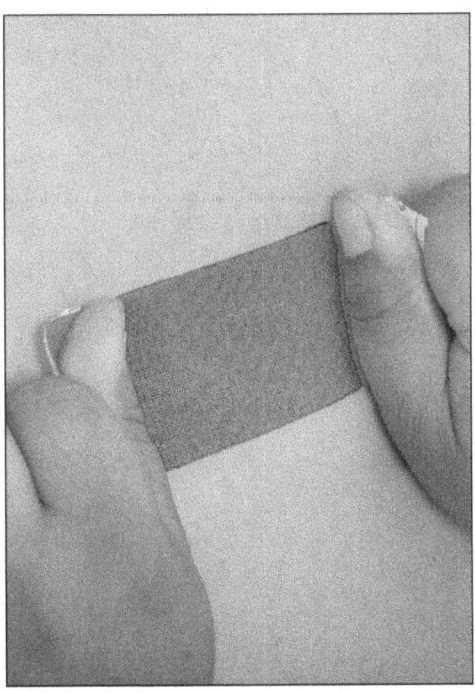

Figure 3.28: Application of strip 1.

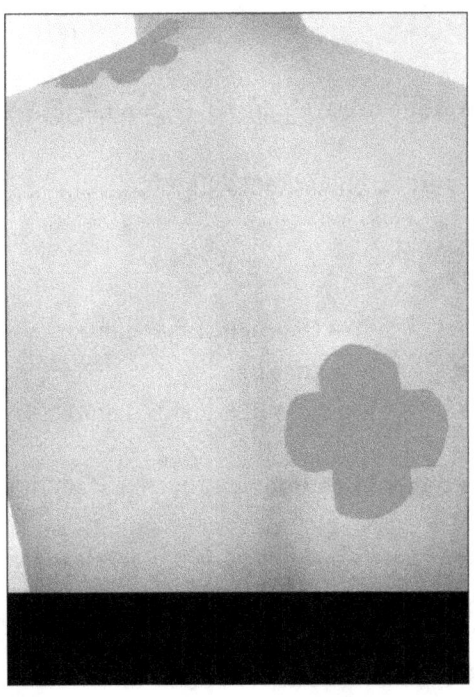

Figure 3.29: Application of strip 2.

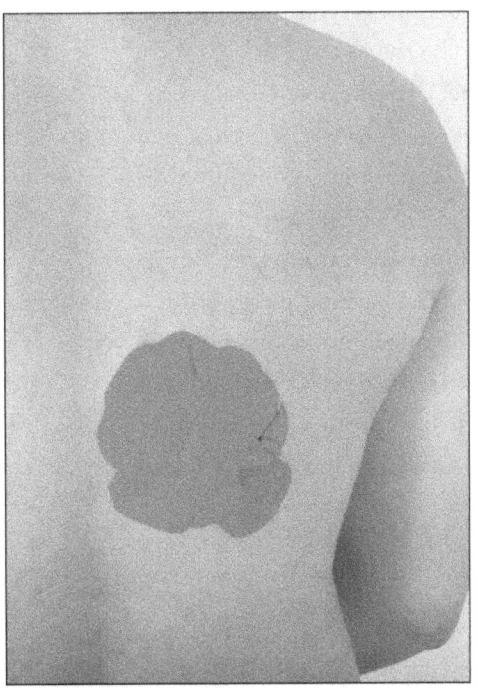

Figure 3.30: Final application of strip.

# Deltoid (Trigger Point)

**Technique used**: Ligament Technique (Space Technique).

**Structure**: Trigger point deltoid[14].

**Indication:**

- Post traumatic rehabilitation.
- Shoulder pain.
- Decrease ROM (abduction).

**Referred pain pattern:** Localized and within 5-10cm.

**Subject position**: Subject sitting in relaxed comfortable position.

**Therapist position**: Therapist standing at the side of the subject.

**Strip**: I-strip is used.

**Procedure:**

- Evaluation: This is the prerequisite of every therapy, the subject must be evaluated and the structure at fault is diagnosed and selection of taping technique is done.
- Part of the subject should be completely clean from dirt and oil and in case of excessive body hair, it should be shaved off.
- Measuring the tape: The subject is asked to keep the joint in neutral and the tape is measured 2cm above and below the area of pain or application.
- Select the required strip design, generally the "I" strip is used in space technique, cut 4 strips of same size.
- The corners of the tapes are rounded off.
- Application of tape: The backing paper of the tape strip is torn from the middle, and the application is just like ligament technique with center of tape is on the pain point while the subject's muscle is in stretched position (Fig: 3.31, Fig: 3.32).
- Apply all the four strips in a plus (+) pattern (Fig: 3.33).
- At the end of application rub the tape until the warmth is felt, this is necessary to activate the glue.

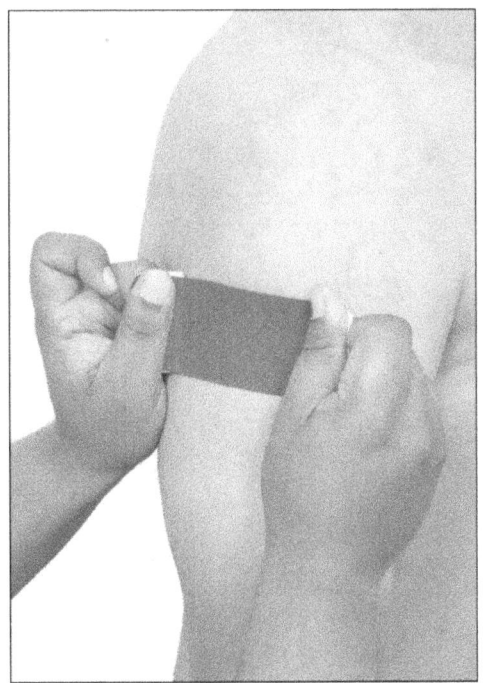

Figure3.31: Application of strip 1.

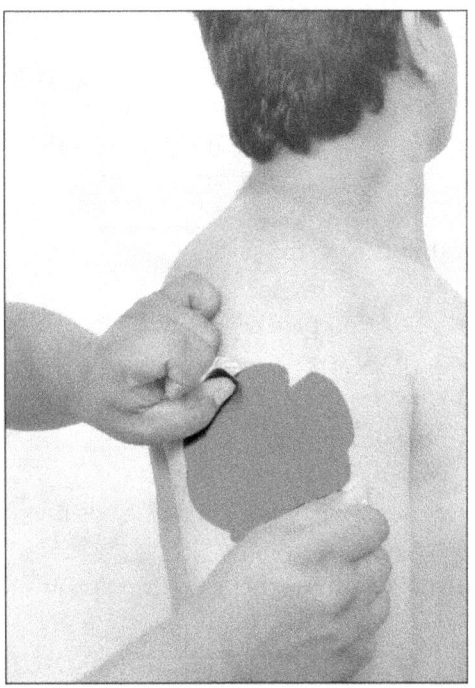

Figure 3.32:  Application of strips.

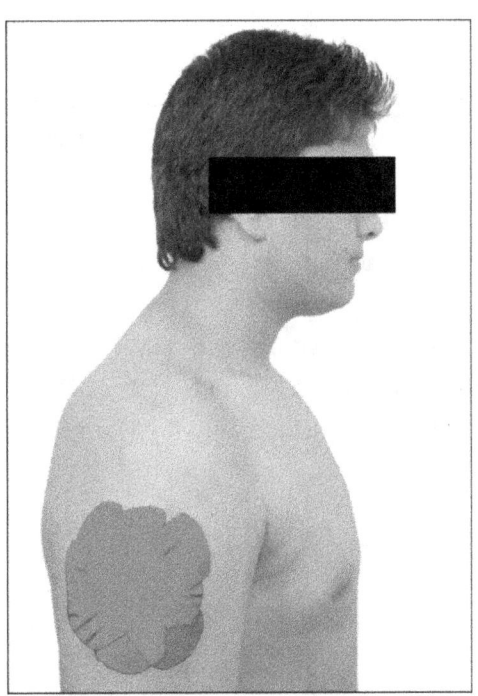

Figure3.33: Final application of strip.

## Lateral Head Gastronemius (Trigger Point)

**Technique used**: Ligament Technique (Space Technique).

**Structure**: Trigger point lateral head gastronemius[45].

**Indication:**

- Calf pain & stiffness.
- Nocturnal cramps.

**Referred pain pattern:** Localize trigger point pain and nearby 5-10cm patch.

**Subject position**: Subject in prone position.

**Therapist position**: Therapist standing at side of the subject.

**Strip**: I-strip is used.

**Procedure:**

- Evaluation : This is the prerequisite of every therapy, the subject must be evaluated and the structure at fault is diagnosed and selection of taping technique is done
- Part of the subject should be completely clean from dirt and oil and in case of excessive body hair, it should be shaved off.
- Measuring the tape:  The subject is asked to keep the joint in neutral and the tape is measured 2cm above and below the area of pain or application.
- Select the required strip design, generally the "I" strip is used in space technique, cut 4 strips of same size.
- The corners of the tapes are rounded off.
- Application of tape: The backing paper of the tape strip is torn from the middle, and the application is just like ligament technique with center of tape is on the pain point while the subject's muscle is in stretched position (Fig: 3.34, Fig: 3.35).
- Apply all the four strips in a plus (+) pattern (Fig: 3.36).
- At the end of application rub the tape until the warmth is felt, this is necessary to activate the glue.

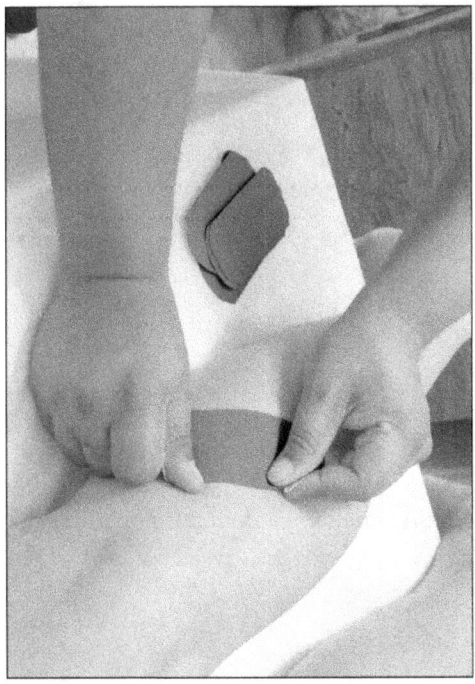

Figure3.34: Application of strip 1.

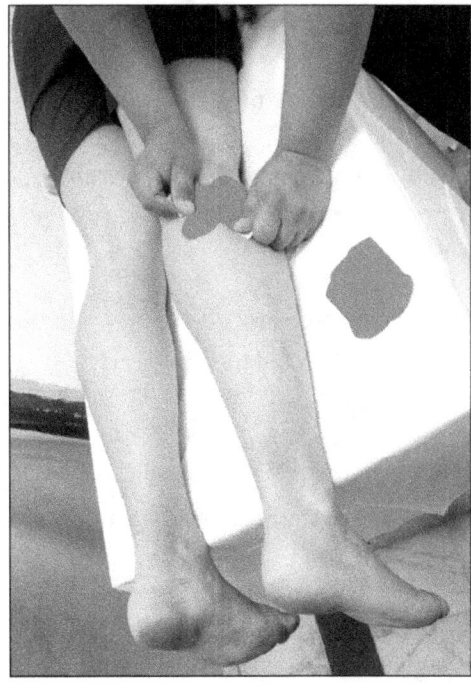

Figure 3.35: Application of strip 2.

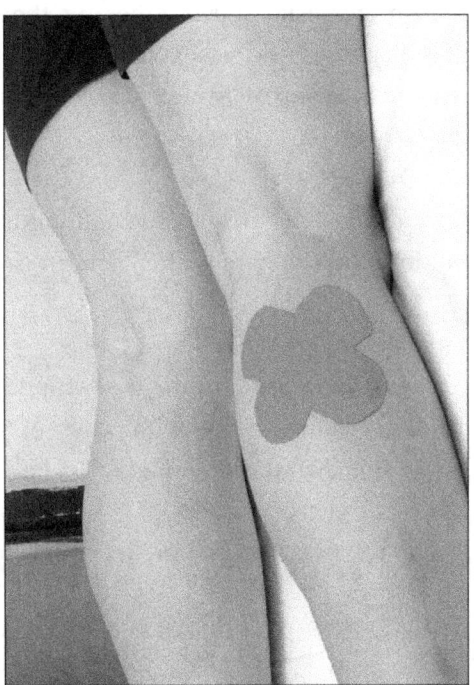

Figure3.36: Final application of strip.

# Tibialis Anterior (Trigger Point)

**Technique used**: Ligament Technique (Space Technique).

**Structure**: Trigger point tibialis anterior [1,9].

**Indication:**

- Ankle pain.
- Pain in big toe (dorsum).
- Shin pain.
- Ankle weakness.

**Referred pain pattern:** Anterio -medial vague pain along with shin zone of 3-5cm of pain on anterior aspect of ankle.

**Subject position**: Subject is in supine lying.

**Therapist position**: Therapist standing at side of the subject.

**Strip**: I-strip is used.

**Procedure:**

- Evaluation : This is the prerequisite of every therapy, the subject must be evaluated and the structure at fault is diagnosed and selection of taping technique is done
- Part of the subject should be completely clean from dirt and oil and in case of excessive body hair, it should be shaved off.
- Measuring the tape:  The subject is asked to keep the joint in neutral and the tape is measured 2cm above and below the area of pain or application.
- Select the required strip design, generally the "I" strip is used in space technique, cut 4 strips of same size.
- The corners of the tapes are rounded off.
- Application of tape: The backing paper of the tape strip is torn from the middle, and the application is just like ligament technique with center of tape is on the pain point while the subject's muscle is in stretched position (Fig: 3.37, Fig: 3.38).
- Apply all the four strips in a plus (+) pattern.
- At the end of application rub the tape until the warmth is felt, this is necessary to activate the glue.

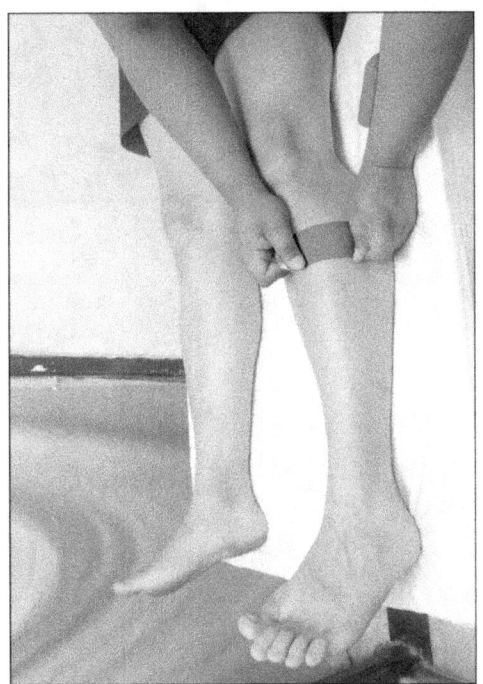

Figure3.37: Application of strip 1.

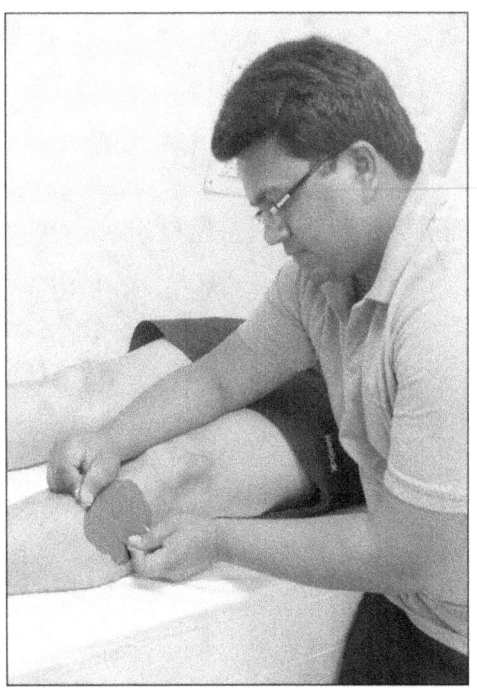

Figure 3.38: Final application of strip.

# CHAPTER 4

# FASCIA & LYMPHATIC CORRECTIVE TECHNIQUES

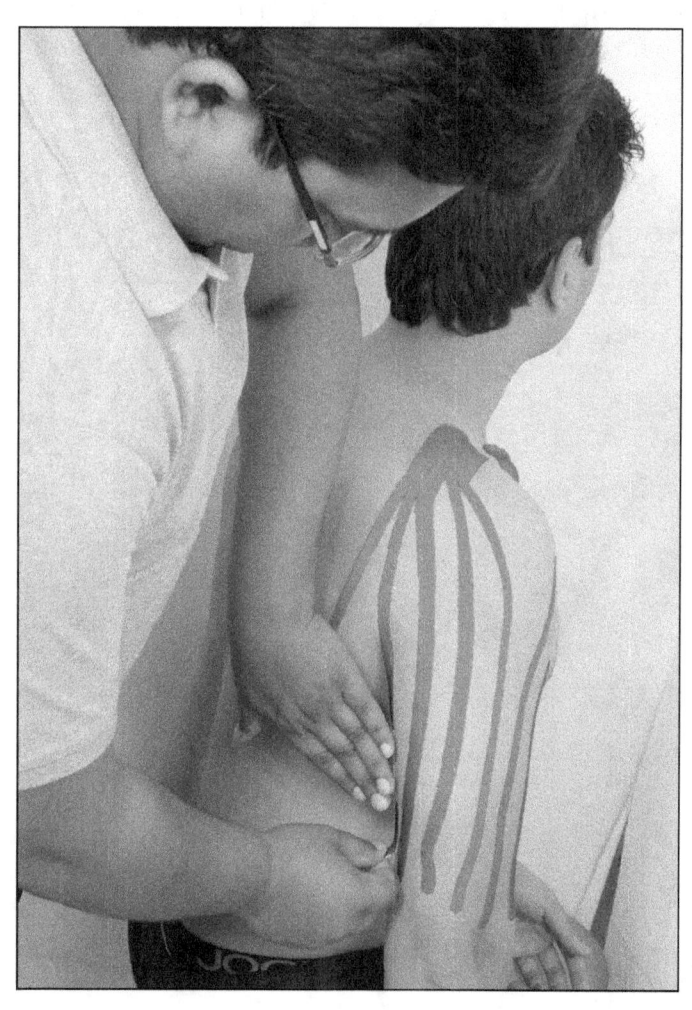

# Fascia Correction Technique

A fascia is a structure of connective tissue that surrounds muscles, groups of muscles, blood vessels, and nerves, binding some structures together, while permitting others to slide smoothly over each other[55,56].

Fasciae are consequently flexible structures that are able to resist great unidirectional tensile forces until the wavy pattern of fibers has been straightened out by the pulling force. The function of muscle fasciae is to reduce friction and to minimize the reduction of muscular force[69].

Myofascial Release is a technique that involves applying gentle sustained pressure into the Myofascial connective tissue restrictions to eliminate pain and restore motion. This essential "time element" has to do with the viscous flow and the piezoelectric phenomenon: a low load (gentle pressure) applied slowly will allow the fascia to elongate[10,49,52].

The kinesiological tape helps to maintain the effects of myofascial release. The tapes can be applied to reposition the fascia and also in conjunction to a manual release. After a manual myofascial release session, the kinesiological tapes can be applied with stretch at center and tails unstretched. The tails are applied with an oscillatory motion while the therapist repositions the fascia manually with hand for desired outcome[22,49].

### Action of the tape

As the base are both the sides and are unstretched while the center of the tape is stretch, the middle will recoil making the base to contract towards the center, the tape will keep the myofascial release effect of the manual therapy for long time[22].

General steps for Fascia techniques:

- Evaluation: This is the prerequisite of every therapy, the subject must be evaluated and the structure at fault is diagnosed and selection of taping technique is done.
- Part of the subject should be completely clean from dirt and oil and in case of excessive body hair, it should be shaved off.
- Measuring the tape: The subject is asked to keep the joint in neutral and the tape is measured 2 cm above and below the area of pain or application.
- Select the required strip design, for fascial correction, generally Y strips are used.
- The corners of the tapes are rounded off.
- Application of tape: The backing paper of the tape strip is torn from the ends, the base is applied unstretched and the tails are stretched to 50-75% and with oscillating motion and with therapist giving manual release of fascia, the tails are applied. The ends of the tails are applied without stretch.
- At the end of application rub the tape until the warmth is felt, this is necessary to activate the glue.

## Fascia application for back.

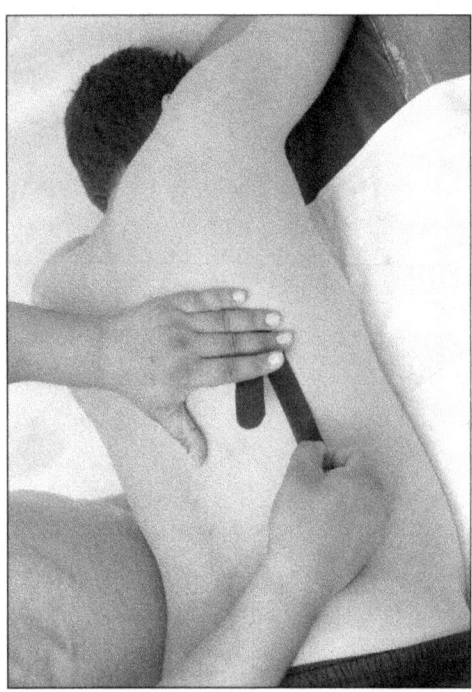

Figure 4.1: Application of base.

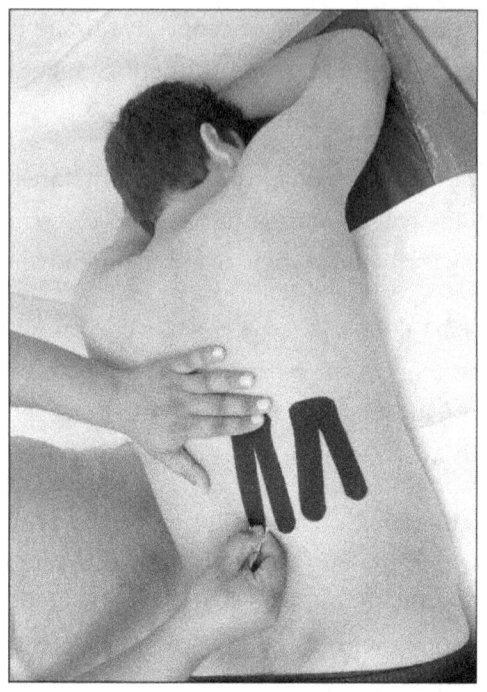

Figure 4.2: Application of second Y strip.

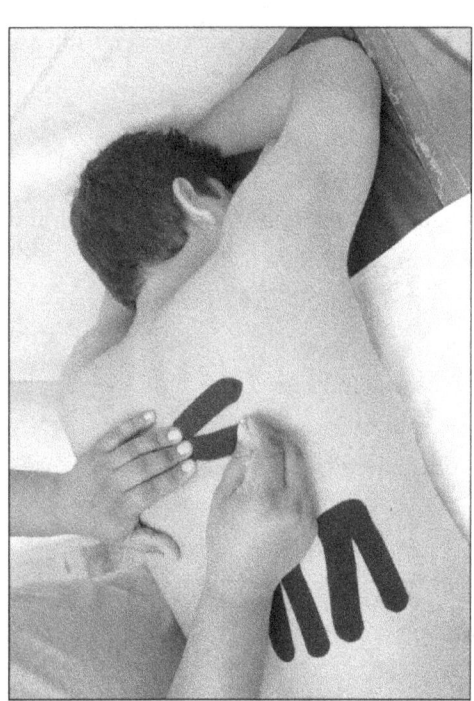

Figure 4.3: Application of tail (2nd application).

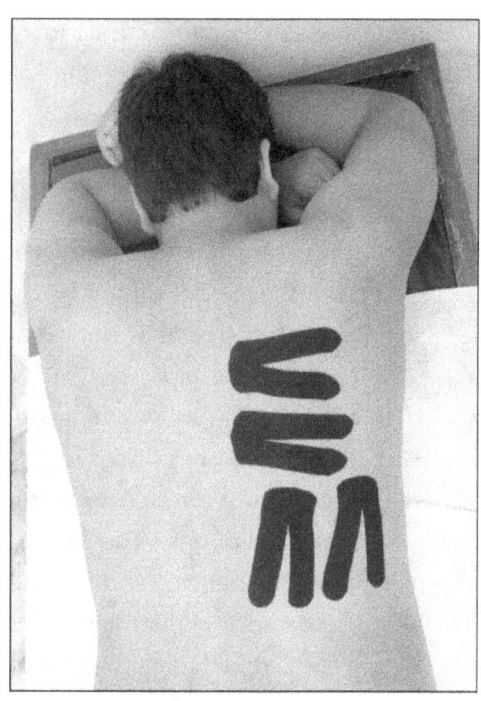

Figure 4.4: Final application.

## Fascia application for thigh.

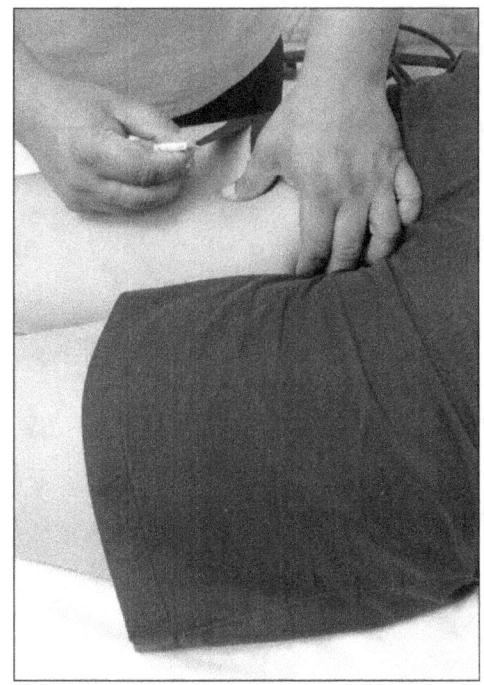

Figure 4.5: Application of Y strip 1.

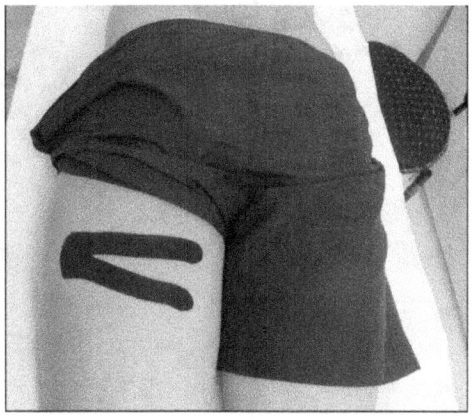

Figure 4.6: Final application 1.

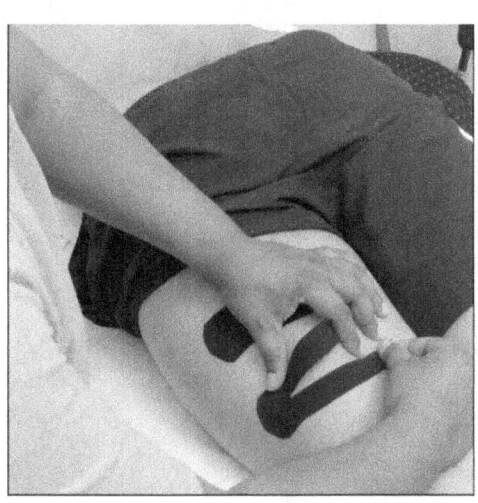

4.7: Application of Y strip 2.

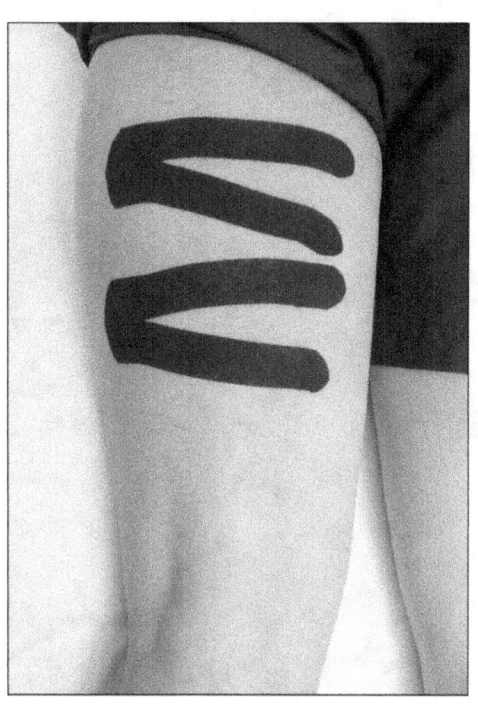

Figure 4.8: Final application.

## Fascia application for leg.

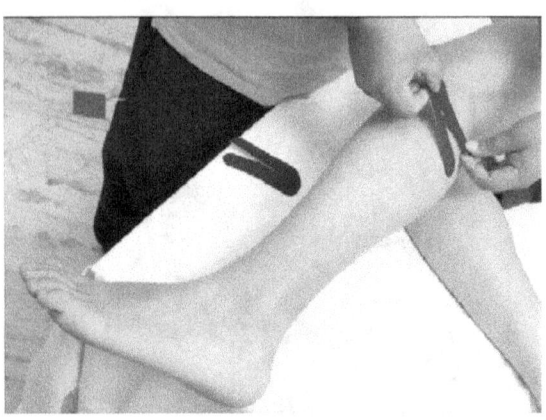

Figure 4.9:Application of Y strip 1.

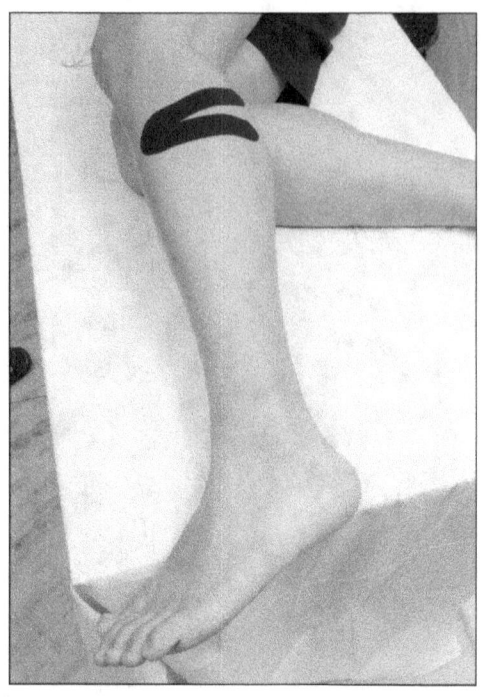

Figure 4.10: Final application 1.

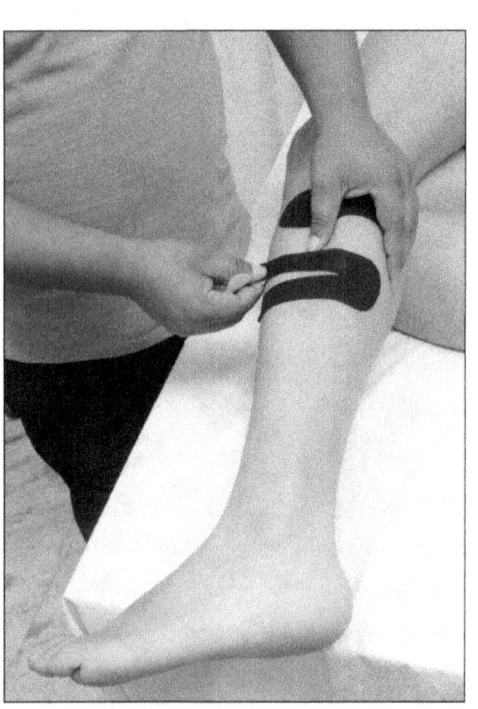

Figure 4.11: Application of Y strip 2.

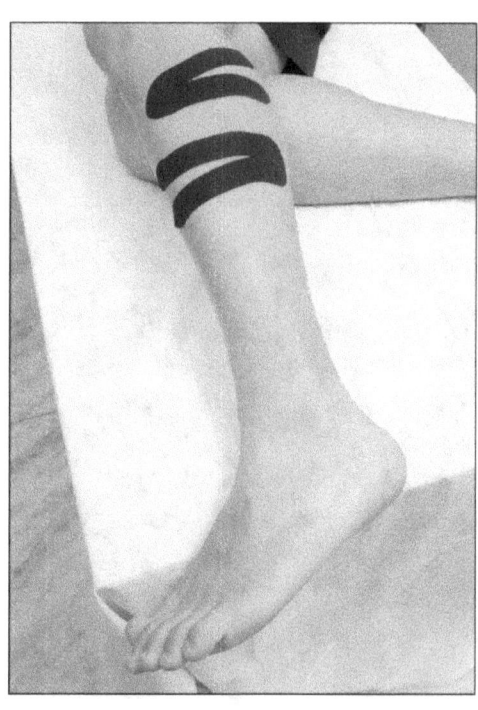

Figure 4.12: Final application 2.

# Lymphatic Correction

The lymphatic system is a part of the circulatory system, comprising a network of conduits called lymphatic vessels that carry a clear fluid called lymph. The lymphatic organs play an important role in the immune system, the blood does not directly come in contact with the parenchymal cells and tissues in the body, but constituents of the blood first exit the microvascular exchange blood vessels to become interstitial fluid, which come into contact with the parenchymal cells of the body[30]. Lymph is the fluid that is formed when interstitial fluid enters the initial lymphatic vessels of the lymphatic system.[30] The lymph is then moved along the lymphatic vessel network by either intrinsic contractions of the lymphatic passages or by extrinsic compression of the lymphatic vessels via external tissue forces. Eventually, the lymph vessels empty into the lymphatic ducts, which drain into one of the two subclavian veins (near the junctions of the subclavian veins with the internal jugular veins)[4].

Lymphedema may be inherited (primary) or caused by injury to the lymphatic vessels (secondary). It is most frequently seen after lymph node dissection, surgery and/or radiation therapy, in which damage to the lymphatic system is caused during the treatment of cancer, most notably breast cancer. Lymphedema may also be associated with accidents or certain diseases or problems that may inhibit the lymphatic system from functioning properly[4].

The kinesiological tapes helps greatly is reduction of lymphedema[30]. The tapes are applied in a fan cut shape with the base near the regional lymph nodes and the strips are applied distally to it. It can also be used to reduce edema caused due to venous insufficiency. Kinesiology tapes have shown great results in treating lymphedema in post-operative cares of breast cancer[30].

**Action of tape:**

The stretchability of tape pulls the skin up creating the space below the skin, which help in reducing the pressure and increase in activity of lymphatic system. The application of tape for 3-4 days repeatedly over 15 days helps in relieving the edema. The wave pattern of the glue not only sticks to skin better but provides a micro massage effect on the skin which helps in increasing the circulation and decreasing the congestion of the fluids[30].

General steps for ligament techniques:

- Evaluation: This is the prerequisite of every therapy, the subject must be evaluated and the structure at fault is diagnosed and selection of taping technique is done.
- Part of the subject should be completely clean from dirt and oil and in case of excessive body hair, it should be shaved off.
- Measuring the tape: The subject is asked to keep the joint in neutral and the tape is measured 2 cm above and below the area of application.
- Select the required strip design , generally the "I" strip are used which is then cut into Fan strips of 4 or 6 strips; depending on the area multiple fan strips can be used for treatment.
- The corners of the tapes are rounded off.
- Application of tape: The backing paper of the tape strip is torn, and the tape is applied depending on the area of application.

- At the end of application rub the tape until the warmth is felt, this is necessary to activate the glue.

## Upper trunk lymphatic correction technique

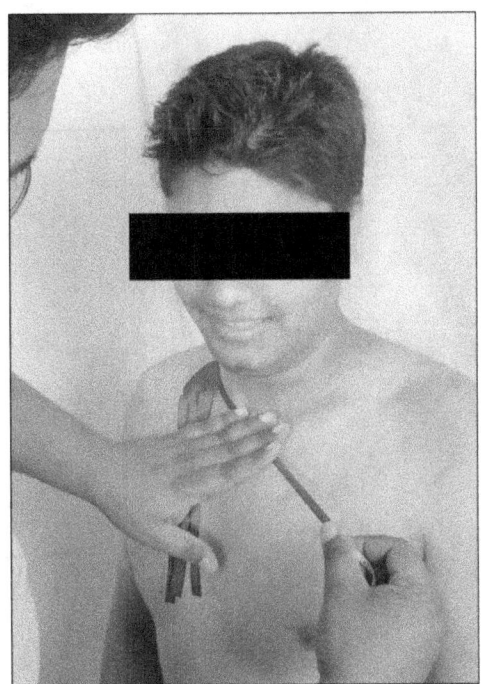

Figure 4.13: Application of base.

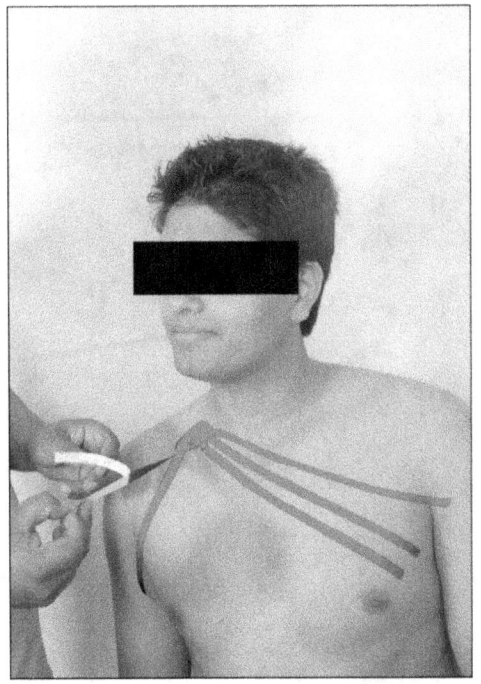

Figure 4.14: Application of fan strips.

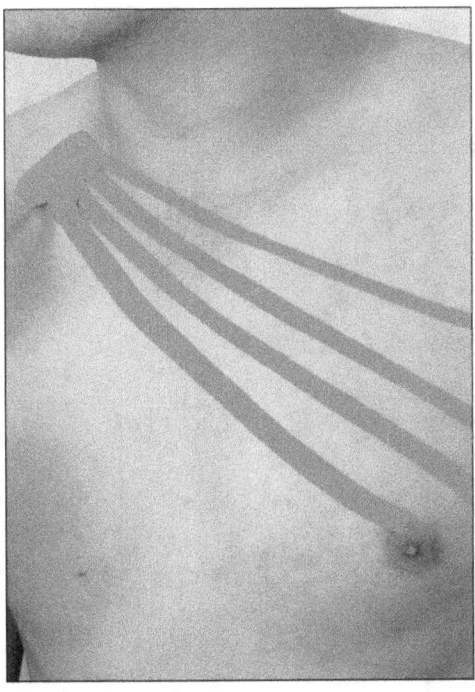

Figure 4.15: Application of fan strips.

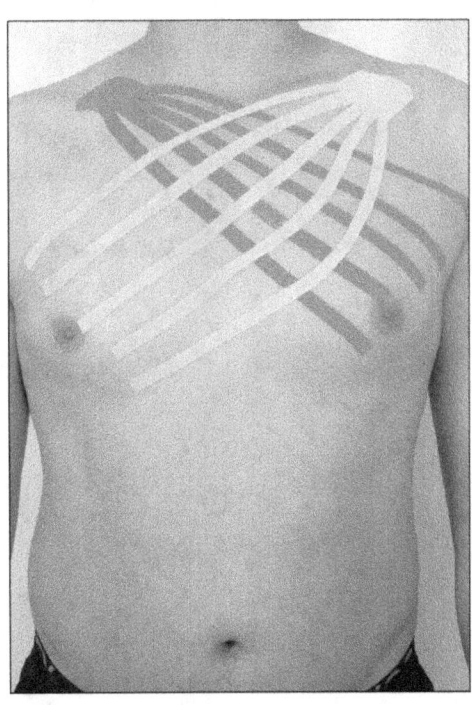

Figure 4.16: Final application of fan strips.

## Shoulder and arm lymphatic correction technique

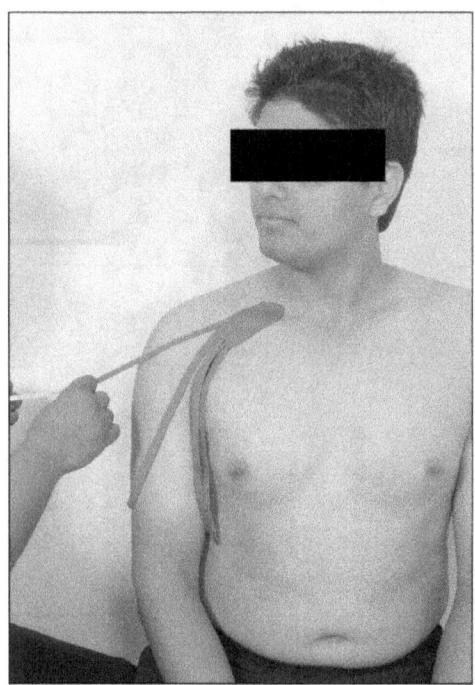

Figure 4.17: Application of base.

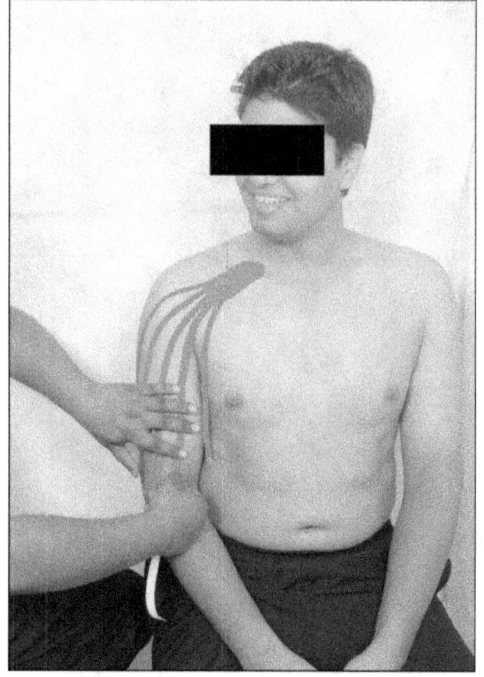

Figure 4.18: Application of fan strips.

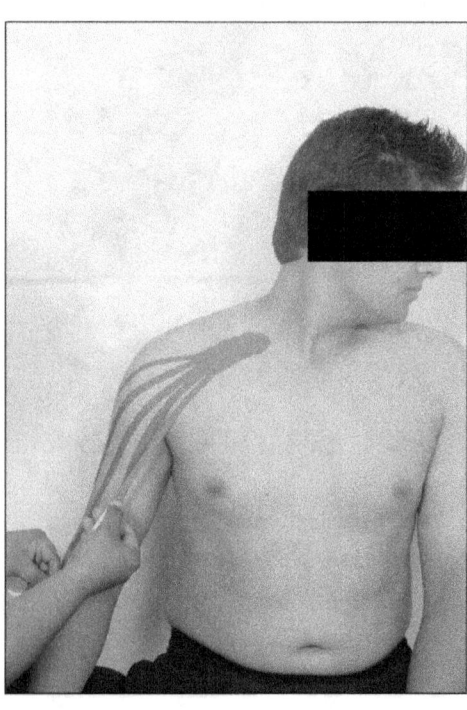

Figure 4.19: Application of fan strips.

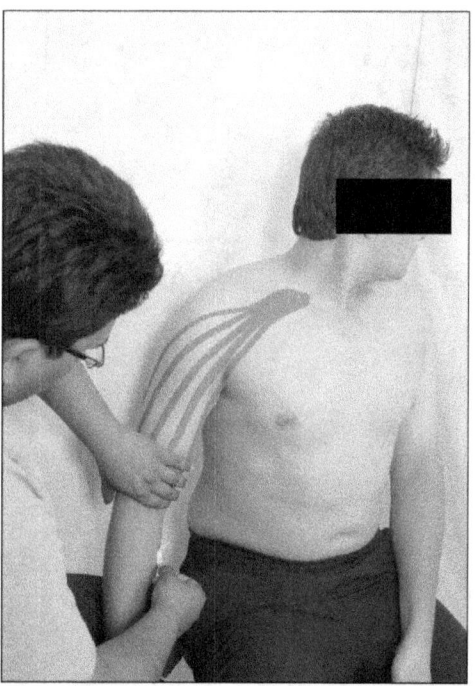

Figure 4.20: Final application of fan strips.

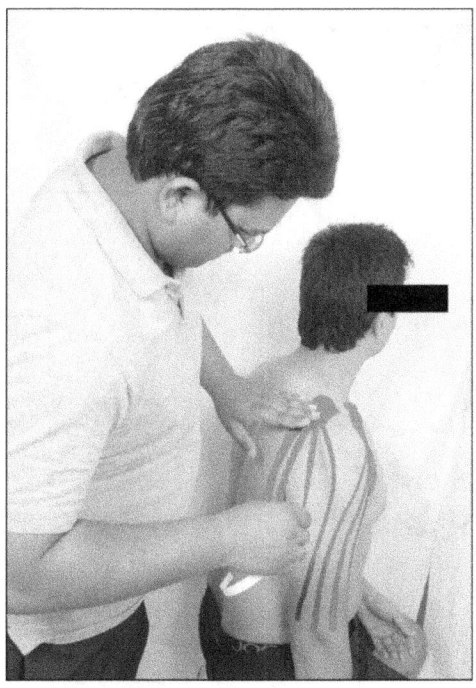

Figure 4.21: Application of fan strips.

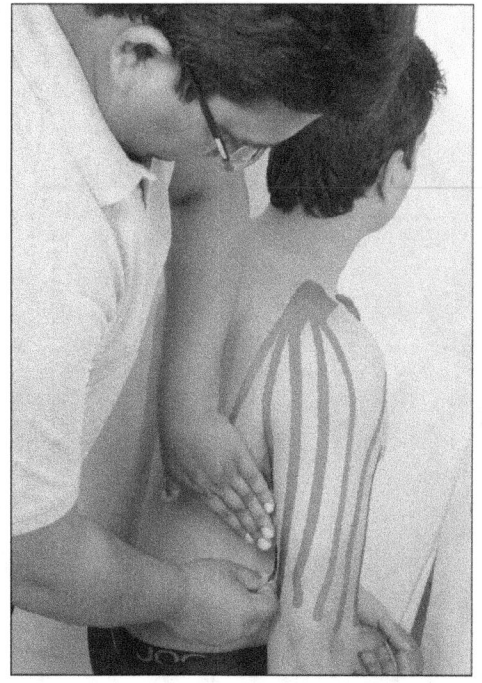

Figure 4.22: Application of fan strips.

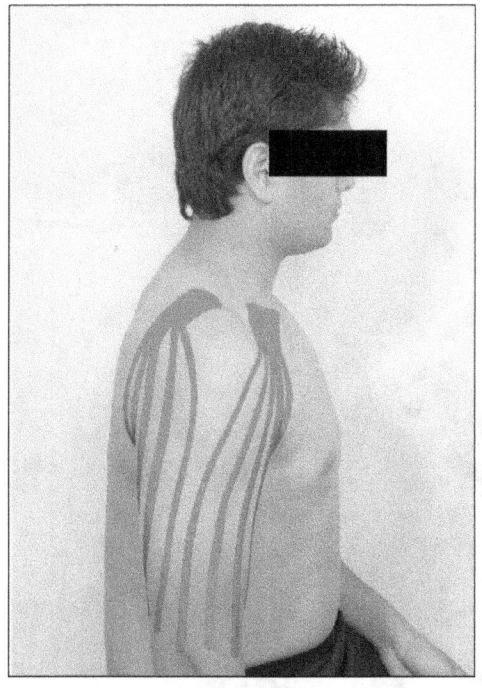

Figure 4.23: Final application of fan strips.

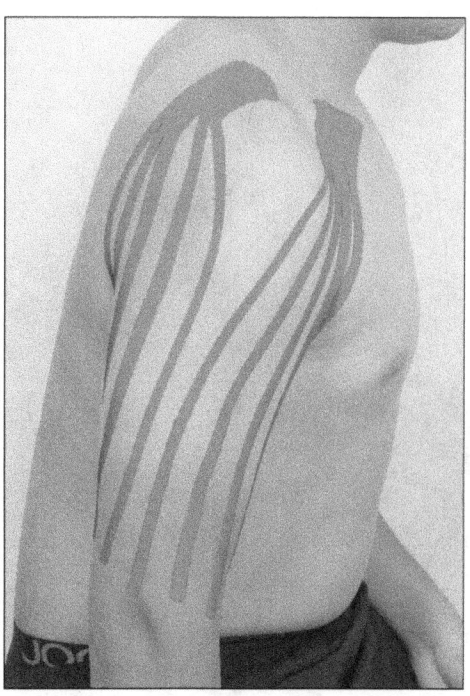

Figure 4.24: Final application of fan strips.

## Forearm and hand lymphatic correction technique

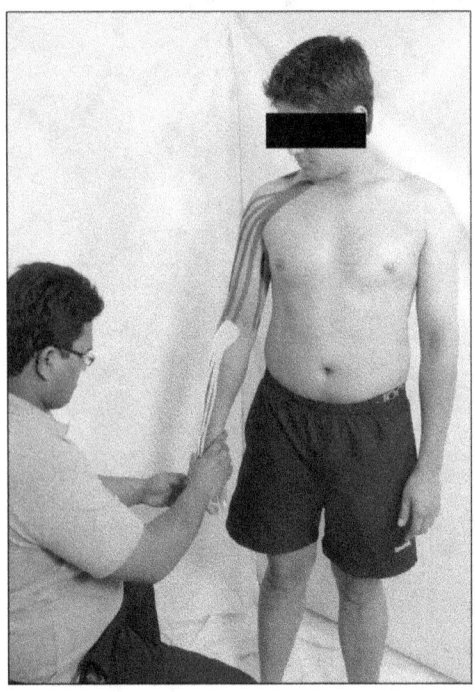

Figure 4.25: Application of fan strips.

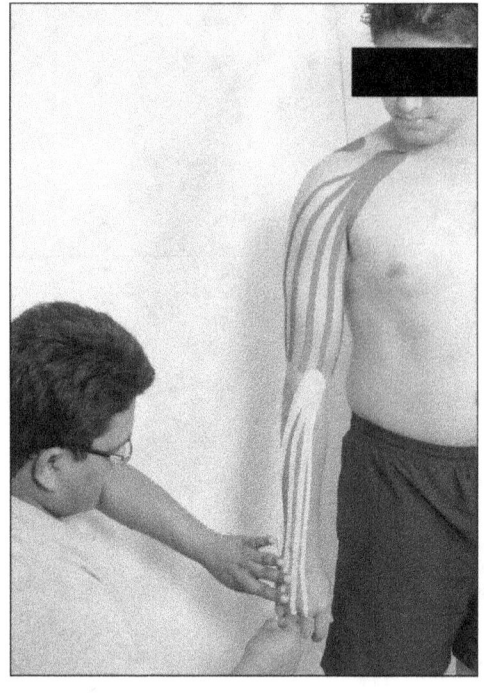

Figure 4.26: Application of fan strips.

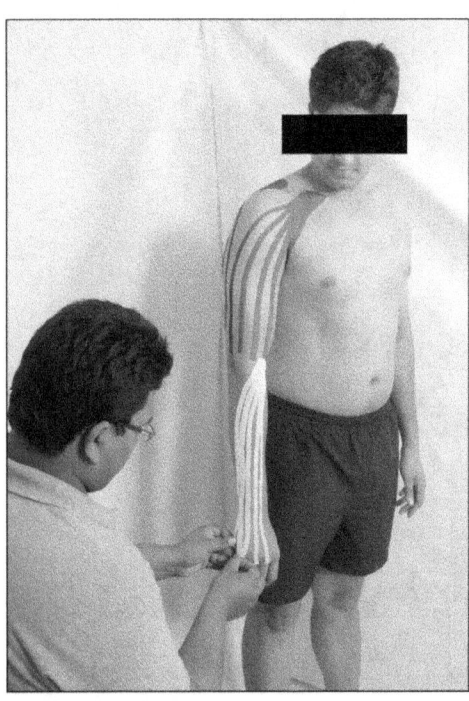

Figure 4.27: Application of fan strips.

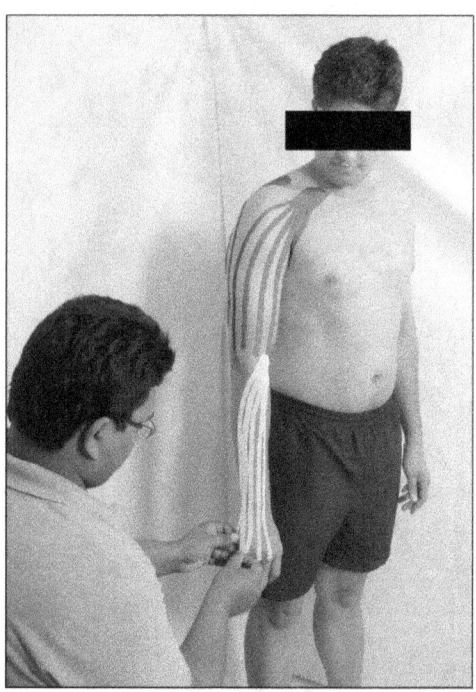

Figure 4.28: Application of fan strips.

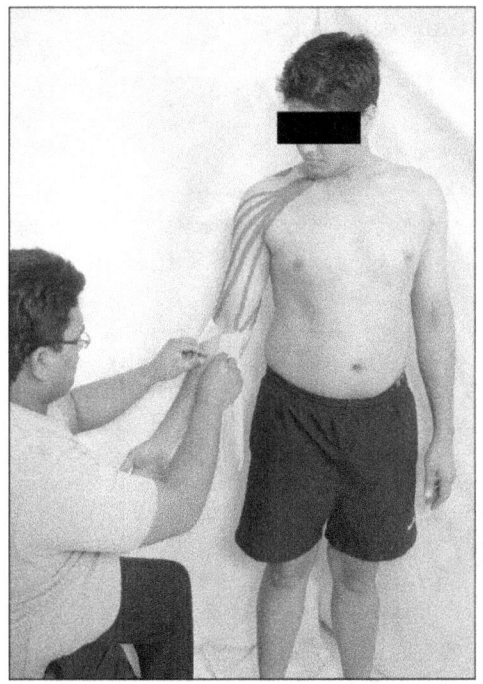

Figure 4.29: Application of fan strips.

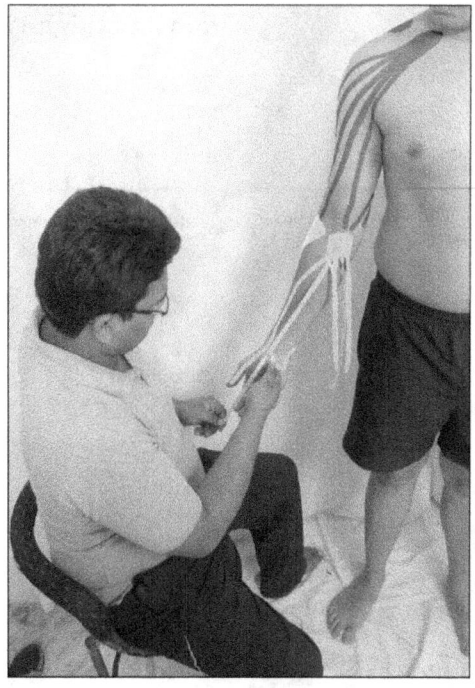

Figure 4.30: Application of fan strips.

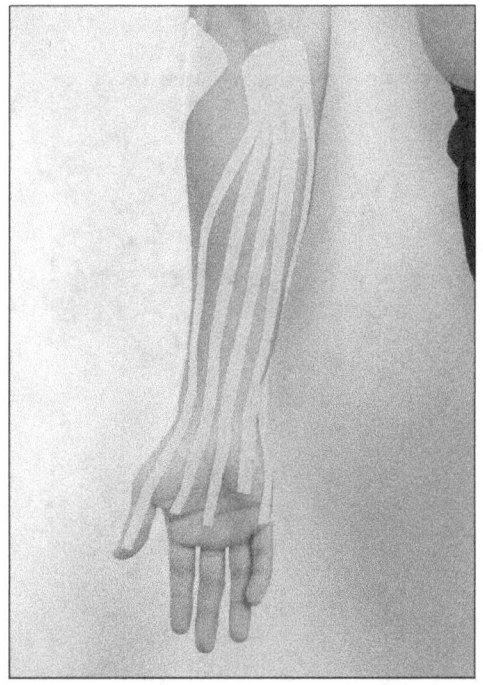

Figure 4.31: Final application of fan strips.

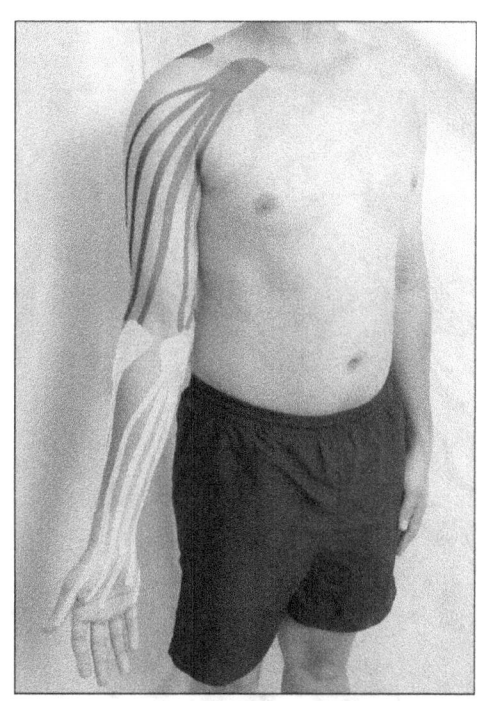

Figure 4.32: Final application of fan strips.

## Groin and thigh lymphatic correction technique

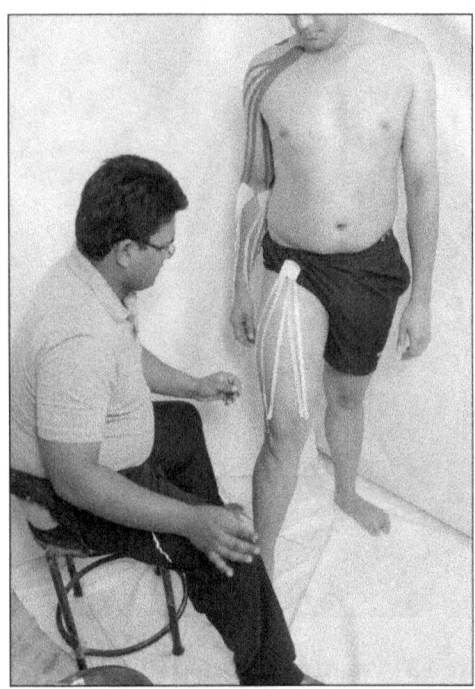

Figure 4.33: Base application of fan strips.

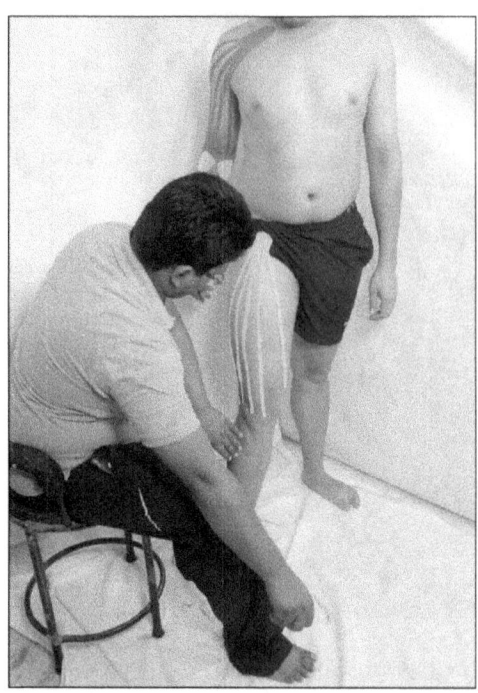

Figure 4.34: Application of fan strips.

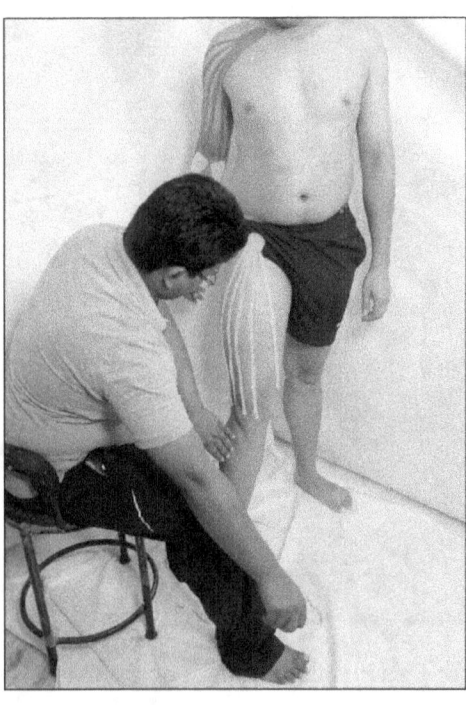

Figure 4.35: Final application of fan strips.

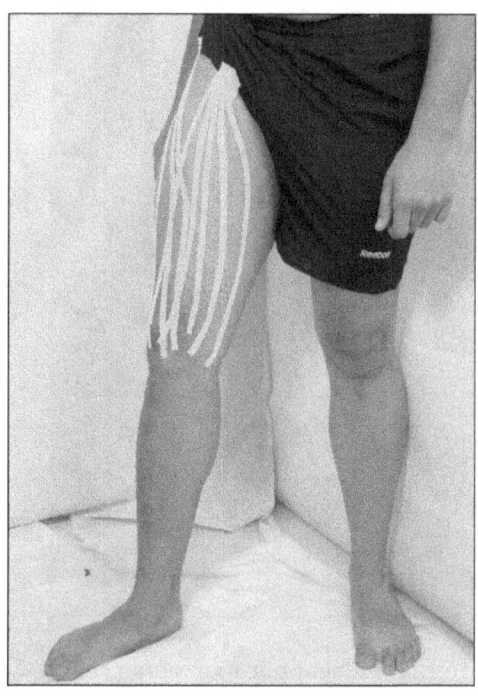

Figure 4.36: Final application of fan strips.

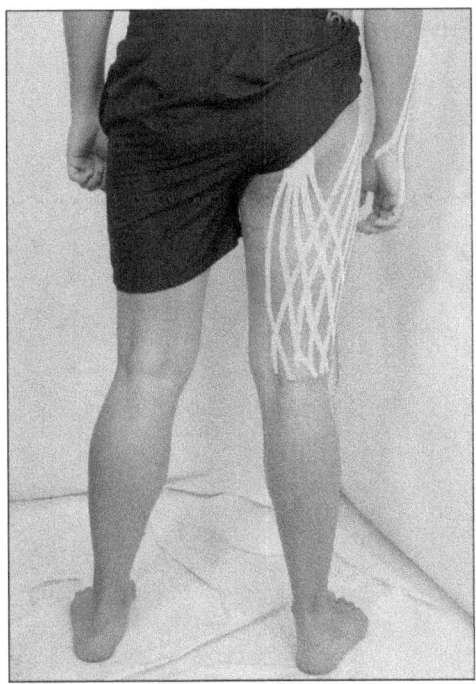

Figure 4.37: Final application of fan strips.

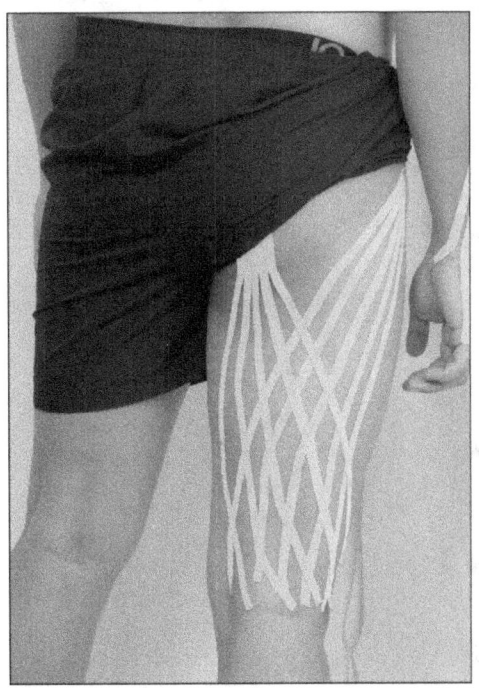

Figure 4.38: Final application of fan strips.

## Calf and foot lymphatic correction technique

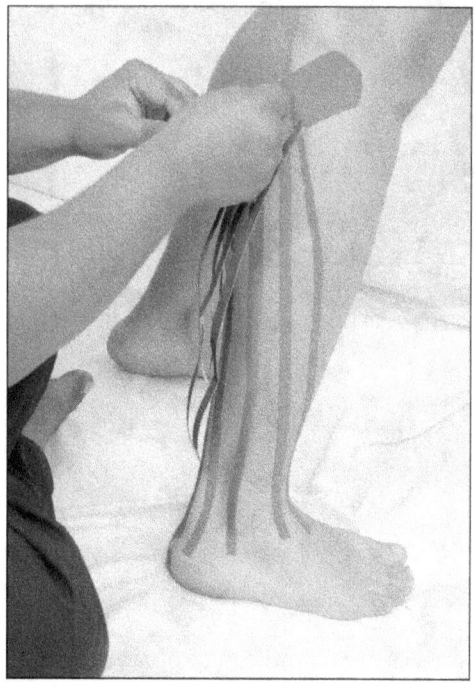

Figure 4.39: Base application of fan strips.

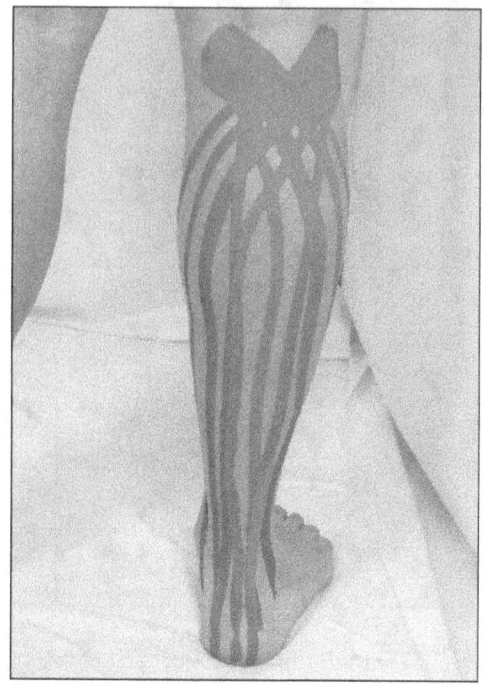

Figure 4.40: Application of fan strips.

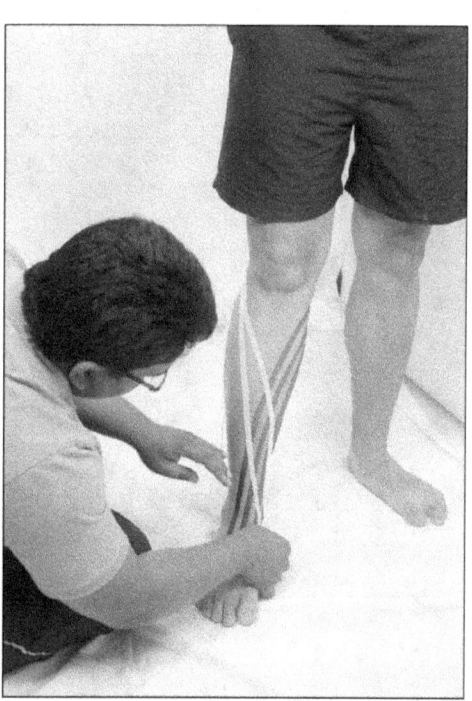

Figure 4.41: Application of fan strips.

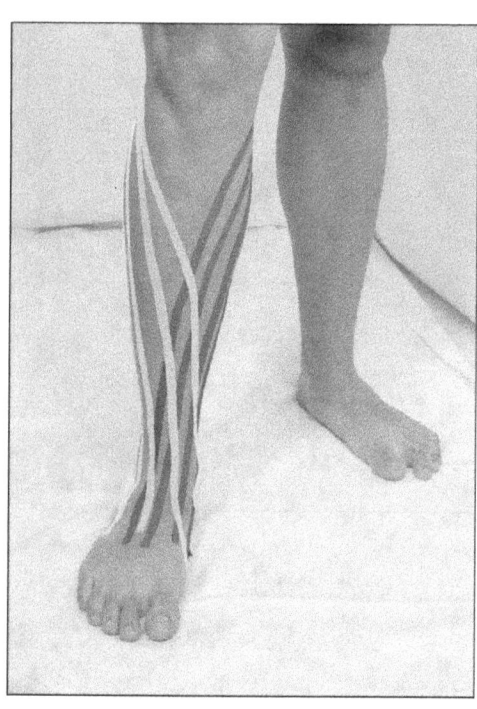

Figure 4.42: Final application of fan strips.

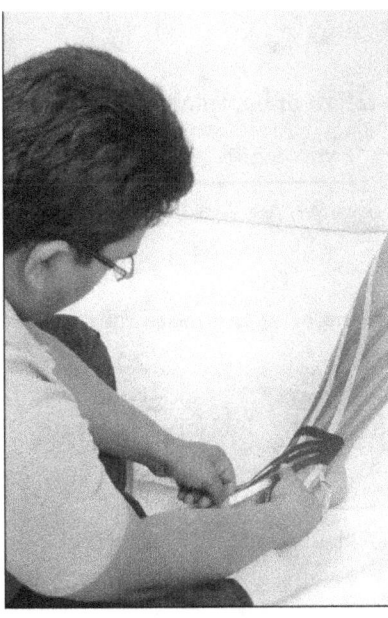

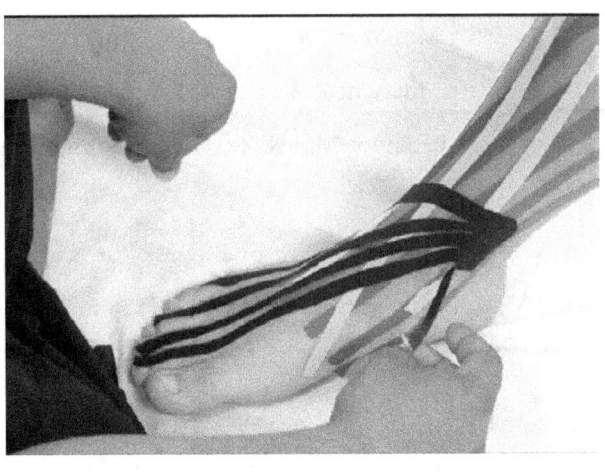

Figure 4.43: Base application of fan strips.

Figure 4.44: Application of fan strips.

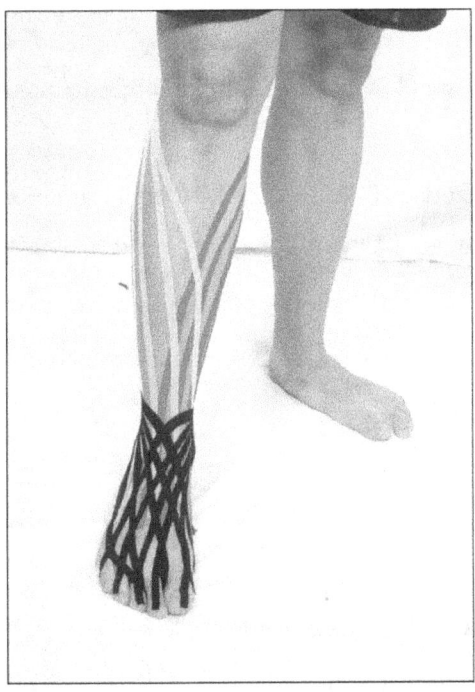

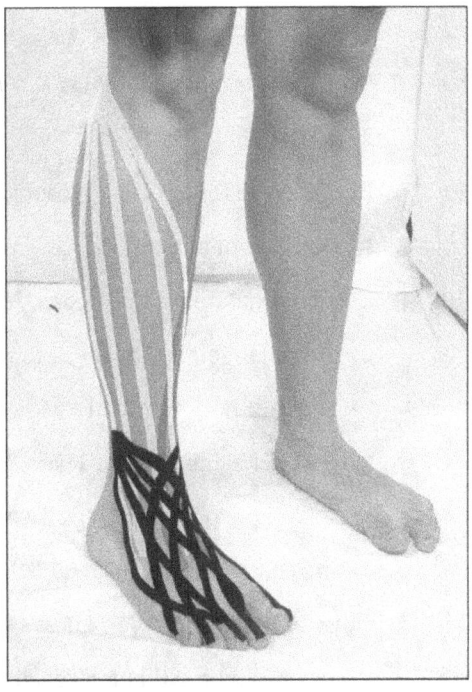

Figure 4.45: Application of fan strips.

Figure 4.46: Final application of fan strips.

# References

1. A.M. Omari, A.S. Lee, S.W. Parsons: The clinical presentation of chronic tibialis anterior insufficiency. Ori R Article Foot and Ankle Sur 1999:Vol 5, Issue 4: 251-259.

2. Alexander Mauskop: Trigeminal neuralgia. J Pain and Sym Mgmt, 1993, Vol 8: Issue 3: 148-154.

3. Anand Nene, Ruth Mayagoitia, Peter Veltink: Assessment of rectus femoris function during initial swing phase. J Gait & Posture, March 1999, Volume 9: 1-9.

4. Anne Williams: Breast and trunk oedema after treatment for breast cancer. J Lymphoedema, Oct 2006: Vol 1, No. 1.

5. B Vicenzino: Lateral epicondylalgia: A musculoskeletal physiotherapy perspective. J Man Th, 2003: Vol 8: 66-79.

6. B. Vicenzino: Manual therapy treatment of tennis elbow. J Sci Med Sports, January 2009: Volume 12.

7. Ben-HuaLuo, Jing-xian Han Cervical Spondylosis Treated by Acupuncture Combined with Movement Therapy. J Trad Chinese Med, June 2010: Vol 30, 2: 113-117.

8. Bradley A. Palmer, Thomas B. Hughes: Cubital Tunnel Syndrome. Jof Hand Sur, January 2010: Vol 35, 1: 153-163.

9. Bryan M. Trout, Gary Hosey, Stuart J. Wertheimer: Rupture of the tibialis anterior tendon. J Foot and Ankle Sur, January 2000:Vol 39, 1: 54-58.

10. César Fernández de lasPeñas, Mónica Sohrbeck Campo, Josué Fernández Carnero, Juan Carlos Miangolarra: Manual therapies in myofascial trigger point treatment: a systematic review. J of Bodywork and Movement Th , January 2005: Vol9, 1: 27-34.

11. Chen-Yu Huang, Tsung-Hsun Hsieh,1 Szu-Ching Lu, and Fong-Chin Su: Effect of the Kinesio tape to muscle activity and vertical jump performance in healthy inactive people. Biomed Eng Online. 2011; 10: 70.

12. Chien-Tsung Tsai, Wen-Dien Chang, Jen-Pei Lee: Effects of Short-term Treatment with Kinesiotaping for Plantar Fasciitis. J Musculoskeletal Pain, March 2010:Vol. 18, No. 1: 71-80.

13. Clement Richard Hanlon :DeQuervain's disease. The Am J of Sur, April 1949: Vol 77, 4: 491-498.

14. Damian M. Rispoli, George S. Athwal, John W. Sperling, Robert H. Cofield: The anatomy of the deltoid insertion. J of Sh and ElbSur,May 2009: Vol 18, 3: 386-390.

15.  David M. Kalainov, Peter E. Hoepfner, Brian J. Hartigan, Charles Carroll IV, James Genuario: Nonsurgical Treatment of Closed Mallet Finger Fractures. Th J of Hand Sur,May 2005: Vol 30, 3: 580-586.

16.  Diana J. Osterhues: The use of Kinesio Taping in the management of traumatic patella dislocation-A case study PhyTh and Prac,2004, 20: 267270.

17.  Dominique Laron, Sanjum P. Samagh, Xuhui Liu, Hubert T. Kim, Brian T. Feeley: Muscle degeneration in rotator cuff tears. J of Sh and Elbow Sur, 2012: Vol 21, 2: 164-174.

18.  Donald B. Slocum: The shin splint syndrome: Medical aspects and differential diagnosis. The Am J of Sur, December 1967: Vol 114, 6: 875-881.

19.  Douglas H. Richie Jr.: Functional instability of the ankle and the role of neuromuscular control. The J of Foot and Ankle Sur, August 2001:Vol 40, 4: 240-251.

20.  Dr. Med. Willem Evermann: Effects of elastic taping on selected functional impairments of the musculoligament apparatus. Komplementäre Integrative Medi, October 2008: Vol 49, Issue 10: 32–36.

21.  Dylan Morrissey: Proprioceptive shoulder taping. J of Bodywork and Movt The, July 2000: Vol 4, 3: 189-194.

22.  Francisco García-Muro, Ángel L. Rodríguez-Fernández, Ángel Herrero-de-Lucas: Treatment of myofascial pain in the shoulder with Kinesio Taping. J Man Th, June 2010: Vol15, 3: 292-295.

23.  G Mirka, D Kelaher, A Baker, A Harrison, J Davis: Selective activation of the external oblique musculature during axial torque production. Clinical Biomech, April 1997: Vol 12, 3: 172-180.

24.  G. Murrell, T. Bradley, D. Fischer, C. Baldwick Dylan, Morrissey: The effect of taping on the shoulders of AFL football players. J of Sci and Med in Sprt, January 2009: Vol 12.

25.  G.R. Mohan, C. Jayalakshmi, A.L. Meena Devi Cervical spondylosis—a clinical study. Bri HomoeoJ, July 1996: Vol 85, 3: 131-133.

26.  Gak Hwang-Bo and Jung-Hoon Lee: Effects of kinesio taping in a physical therapist with acute low back pain due to patient handling- A case report International J of Occup Med and Enviro Health, 2011, Vol 24, 3:320-323.

27.  Gary C Hunt, Tom Sneed, Herb Hamann, Sheldon Chisam: Biomechanical and histiological considerations for development of plantar fasciitis and evaluation of arch taping as a treatment option to control associated plantar heel pain: a single-subject design. The Foot, September 2004: Vol 14, 3: 147-153.

28. Glenn A. Hebel A case of traumatic temperomandibular joint dislocation The Journal of Emergency Medicine, Volume 13, Issue 6, November–December 1995, Page 803

29. HAC Jacob, RO Kissling: The mobility of the sacroiliac joints in healthy volunteers between 20 and 50 years of age. Clinical biomech, October 1995: Vol 10, 7: 352-361.

30. Han-Ju Tsai, Hsiu-Chuan Hung, Jing-Lan Yang, Chiun- Sheng Huang and Jau-Yih Tsauo: Could Kinesiotape replace the bandage in decongestive lymphatic therapy for breast-cancer-related lymphedema- A pilot study. Supportive Care in Cancer, 2009:Vol 17, 11: 1353-1360.

31. Harold Ellis: Anatomy of the anterior abdominal wall and inguinal canal. Anaes& Intensive Care Medi, July 2009: Vol 10, 7: 315-317.

32. Horace Stimson: Bursitis. The Am J Sur, December 1940: Vol 50, 3: 527-533.

33. Hsiao-Yun Chang, Kun-Yu Chou, Jau-Jia Lin, Chih-Feng Lin, Chun-Hou Wang: Immediate effect of forearm Kinesio taping on maximal grip strength and force sense in healthy collegiate athletes. Phy The Sp, November 2010: Vol 11, 4:122-127.

34. Ilse Jonkers, Caroline Stewart, Kaat Des loovere, Guy Molenaers, Arthur Spaepen: Musculo-tendon length and lengthening velocity of rectus femoris in stiff knee gait. Gait & Posture, February 2006: Vol 23, 2: 222-229.

35. J.D.G. Troup: Biomechanics of the lumbar spinal canal. Clinical Biomech, February 1986: Vol 1, 1: 31-43.

36. J.U. McCarthy Persson, A.C.B. Hooper, H.E. Fleming Repeatability of skin displacement and pressure during "inhibitory" vastus lateralis muscle taping. Manual Th, February 2007: Vol 12, 1: 17-21.

37. Jay D. Keener, DaraChafik, H. Mike Kim, Leesa M. Galatz, Ken Yamaguchi: Insertional anatomy of the triceps brachii tendon. J of Sh and Elbw Sur, April 2010: Vol 19, 3: 399-405.

38. Jeffrey Borkan, Shmuel Reis, Doron Hermoni, Aya Biderman: Talking about the pain - A patient-centered study of low back pain in primary care. Social Sci&Medi, April 1995: Vol40, 7, :977-988.

39. Jenny McConnell, Cyril Donnelly, Samuel Hamner, James Dunne, Thor Besier : Passive and Dynamic Shoulder Rotation Range in Uninjured and Previously Injured Overhead Throwing Athletes and the Effect of Shoulder Taping. PM&R February 2012, Vol 4,2: : 111-116.

40. Jo Nijs, Nathalie Roussel, Kim Vermeulen, Greet Souvereyns Scapular Positioning in Patients With Shoulder Pain -A Study examining the Reliability and Clinical Importance of 3 Clinical Tests. Arch of Phy Medi and Rehab, July 2005: Vol86, 7: 1349-1355.

41. Joanne Middleton: Cervical spondylosis and ossification of the posterior longitudinal ligament - Case report of a Caucasian patient. Clinical Chirop, September 2005: Vol 8, 3: 145-150.

42. John M. McPartland, Raymond R. Brodeur Rectus capitis posterior minor: a small but important sub occipital muscle. J of Bodywork and MovtTh, January 1999: Vol 3, 1: 30-35.

43. Julie Kohls-Gatzoulis, John Angel, Dishan Singh:Tibialis posterior dysfunction as a cause of flatfeet in elderly patients. The Foot, December 2004: Vol 14, 4: 207-209.

44. Jung-hoon Lee, Won-gyuYoo: Application of posterior pelvic tilt taping for the treatment of chronic low back pain with sacroiliac joint dysfunction and increased sacral horizontal angle.PhTh in Sp: 7 Dec 2011.

45. Jung-hoon Lee, Won-gyuYoo: Treatment of chronic Achilles tendon pain by Kinesio taping in an amateur badminton player. Phy Th in Sp: 15 Sept 2011.

46. K Mizobuchi, S Kuwabara, S Toma, Y Nakajima, K Ogawara, T Hattori Properties of human skin mechanoreceptors in peripheral neuropathy. Cli Neurophysiology, February 2002: Vol113, 2,: 310-315.

47. KaratasN, Bicici S, Baltaci G, Caner H: The effect of Kinesiotape application on functional performance in surgeons who have musculo-skeletal pain after performing surgery. Turk Neurosurg. 2012: 22, 1:83-9.

48. Kohei Hasegawa, Joel M. Schofer Rupture of the Pectoralis Major: A Case Report and Review Original Research Article The J of Emergency Medi, February 2010: Vol38, 2:196-200

49. Le Bauer A, Brtalik R, Stowe K: The effect of myofascial release (MFR) on an adult with idiopathic scoliosis. Jof Bodywork and movt Th, 2008Oct: 12 :4:356-63.

50. Lee Herrington: The effect of patella taping on quadriceps strength and functional performance in normal subjects. Phy Th in Sp, February 2004: Vol 5, 1: 33-36.

51. Lee Herrington, Sharon Malloy, Jim Richards: The effect of patella taping on vastus medialis oblique and vastus laterialis EMG activity and knee kinematic variables during stair descent. J of Electromyography and Kinesiology, December 2005: Vol15, 6: 604-607.

52. Leonid Kalichman, Elisha Vered, Lior Volchek: Relieving Symptoms of Meralgia Paresthetica Using Kinesio Taping - A Pilot Study, Arch of Phy Medi and Rehab, July 2010: Vol 91, 7: 1137-1139

53. Luke D. Rickards: The effectiveness of non-invasive treatments for active myofascial trigger point pain - A systematic review of the literature. J of Osteop Medi, December 2006: Vol 9, 4: 120-136.

54. M. Christopher McGrath: Palpation of the sacroiliac joint: An anatomical and sensory challenge International J Osteop Med, September 2006: Vol 9, 3: 103-107.

55. M.S. Ajimsha, SaraladeviChithra, Ramiah Pillai Thulasyammal: Effectivenes Myofascial Release in the Management of Lateral Epicondylitis in Computer Professionals. Arch of Physical Medi and Rehab, 10 January 2012.

56. Maria Adele Giamberardino, Giannapia Affaitati, Alessandra Fabrizio, Raffaele Costantini Myofascial pain syndromes and their evaluation. Best Practice & Research Clinical Rheumatology, April 2011: Vol 25, 2: 185-198.

57. Matthew E. Alix, Deanna K. Bates: A proposed etiology of cervicogenic headache- The neurophysiologic basis and anatomic relationship between the dura mater and the rectus posterior capitis minor muscle. J of Manip and Physiological Therap, October 1999: Vol 22, 8: 534-539.

58. Mc McGrath: Clinical considerations of sacroiliac joint anatomy- A review of function, motion and pain. J Osteopath Med , April 2004: Vol 7, 1: 16-24.

59. Megan Drakeley, Jennie Long bottom A single case report of physiotherapy and acupuncture treatment for cervical radiculopathy European Journal of Integrative Medicine, In Press, Corrected Proof, Available online 11 February 2012

60. Menno Braakman, Esther E. Oderwald, Marleen H.H.J. Haentjens: Functional taping of fractures of the 5th metacarpal results in a quicker recovery. Article Inj, January 1998 : Vol 29, 1: 5-9.

61. Michael J. Callaghan, James Selfe, Alec McHenry, Jacqueline A. Oldham: Effects of patellar taping on knee joint proprioception in patients with patellofemoral pain syndrome. M Th, June 2008: Vol 13, 3: 192-199.

62. Michael O. Egwu, Benjamin A. Ajao, Chidozie E. Mbada, Isaac O. Adeoshun: Isometric Grip Strength and Endurance of Patients With Cervical Spondylosis and Healthy Controls- A Comparative Study: Hong Kong Physio J 2009, Vol 27, 1: 2-6.

63. Michael R. Boland, Tracy Spigelman, Tim L. Uhl: The Function of Brachioradialis. The J of Hand S, December 2008: Vol 33, 10: 1853-1859.

64. Michael Smith, Valerie Sparkes, Monica Busse, Stephanie Enright: Upper and lower trapezius muscle activity in subjects with subacromial impingement symptoms- is there imbalance and can taping change it. Clinics in Sp Med : July 2001: Vol 20, 3: 621–639.

65. N.A. Segal, N.A. Glass, J. Torner, M. Yang, D.T. Felson, L. Sharma, M. Nevitt, C.E. Lewis. Quadriceps weakness predicts risk for knee joint space narrowing in women in the mostcohort. Art Osteoarthritis and Cart: June 2010: Vol 18, 6: 769-775.

66. Nicholas WM Thomas: Low-back pain, sciatica, cervical and lumbar spondylosis. Article Surgery: Vol 22, 2, 1 February 2004: 25-28.

67. Nikolai Bogduk: The anatomy and pathophysiology of whiplash. Clinical Biomechanics, May 1986: Vol 1, 2: 92-101.

68. Oluwaleke Sokunbi, Vinette Cross, Peter Watt, Ann Moore: Experiences of individuals with chronic low back pain during and after their participation in a spinal stabilisation exercise programme – A pilot qualitative study. Article M Th, April 2010: Vol 15, 2: 179-184.

69. P. Prithvi Raj, Lee Ann Paradise: Myofascial pain syndrome and its treatment in low back pain. Sem in Pain Med, September 2004: Vol4 ,3 : 167-174.

70. Paoloni M, Bernetti A, Fratocchi G, Mangone M, Parrinello L, Del Pilar Cooper M, Sesto L, Di Sante L, Santilli V:Kinesio Taping applied to lumbar muscles influences clinical and electromyographic characteristics in chronic low back pain patients. Eur J Phys Rehabil Med. 2011 Jun:47 Vol2:237-44.

71. R.S. Johansson, U. Landstro¨m, R. Lundstro¨m. Responses of mechanoreceptive afferent units in the glabrous skin of the human hand to sinusoidal skin displacements: Brain Research, 22 July 1982: Vol 244, 1: 17-25.

72. Rajeev Bansal, Chris Taylor, Ashvin L. Pimpalnerkar: Snapping knee- An unusual biceps femoris tendon injury. The Knee, December 2005: Vol 12, 6: 458-460.

73. Robert J. Spinner, Shawn W. O' Driscoll, Jon R. Davids, Richard D. Goldner: Cubitus Varus Associated With Dislocation of Both the Medial Portion of the Triceps and the Ulnar Nerve. The Journal of Hand Surgery, 1999: Vol 24, 4: 718-726.

74. Sandra Mathieu, Clément Prati, Marie Bossert, ÉricToussirot : Acute prepatellar and olecranon bursitis - Retrospective observational study in 46 patients. Joint Bone Spine, 2011 Jul: 78,4: 423-4.

75. Scott Haldeman, Simon Dagenais: Cervicogenic headaches-A critical review. The Spine J, February 2001: Vol 1, 1: 31-46.

76. Şimşek TT, Türkücüoğlu B, Çokal N, Üstünbaş G: The effects of Kinesio taping on sittin posture, functional independence and gross motor function in children with cerebral palsy. Disabil Rehabil. 2011;Vol33: 2058-63.

77. Smith M, Sparkes V, Busse M, Enright S: Upper and lower trapezius muscle activity in subjects with subacromial impingement symptoms- is there imbalance and can taping change it. Phys Ther Sport. 2009 :Vol10,2:45-50.

78. Stephanie H. Hsu, Suzanne L. Miller, Alan S. Curtis: Long Head of Biceps Tendon Pathology-Management Alternatives. Clini in Sp Med, October 2008: Vol 27, 4: 747-762.

79. Steve Iscoe: Control of abdominal muscles. J Prog in Neurobio ,November 1998: Vol56, 4: 433-506.

80. T Saxby: Turf toe. J of Sci and Med in Sp, March 1999: Vol2, 1, : Page 36.

81. T. Bradley Edwards, Gilles Walch: Biceps tenodesis: Indications and techniques.Oper Tech in Sp Med, April 2002: Vol 10, 2: 99-104.

82. Thomas M. Greiner, M. Elizabeth Bedford, Robert A. Walker: Variability in the human M. spinaliscapitis and cervicis: frequencies and definitions. Ann of Anatomy, April 2004: Vol 186, 2: 185-191.

83. Tieh-Cheng Fu, Alice M.K. Wong, Yu-Cheng Pei, Katie P. Wu, Shih-Wei Chou, Yin-Chou Lin: Effect of Kinesio taping on muscle strength in athletes—A pilot study. J Sci and Med in Sp, April 2008 :Vol 11, 2: 198-201.

84. Tim l. uhl, James A. Madaleno: Rehabilitation Concepts And Supportive Devices for Overuse Injuries Of The Upper extremities  Division of Athletic Training.Clin Sports Med. 2001 Jul;20,3: 621-39.

85. Tom Hughes, Patsy Rochester: The effects of proprioceptive exercise and taping on n proprioception in subjects with functional ankle instability- A review of the literature review. Art Phy Th in Sp, August 2008:Vol 9, 3 : 136-147.

86. The effect of a taping technique on pain and range of motion in athelete with shoulder impingement. J Sci and Med Sp, Vol 7,:Issue 4: Dec 2004: 105.

87. Toshikazu Tani, Hiroshi Yamamoto, Masahirolchimiya, Jun Kimura: Reflexes evoked in human erector spinae muscles by tapping during voluntary activity .J Electroencephalography and Clini Neurophysio and Motor Cont, June 1997: Vol 105, 3: 194-200.

88. Vittorio Franco, Guglielmo Cerullo, Enrico Gianni, Giancarlo Puddu :Iliotibial band friction syndrome. OpTech in Sp Med, July 1997: Vol 5, 3: 153-156.

89. Walsh SF: Treatment of a brachial plexus injury using kinesiotape and exercise. Physiother Theory Pract. 2010 Oct;26(7):490-6.

90. Wen-Chi Chen, Wei-Hsien Hong, Tien Fen Huang, Horng-Chaung Hsu: Effects of kinesio taping on the timing and ratio of vastus medialis obliquus and vastus lateralis muscle for person with patellofemoral pain. J of Biomec, 2007: Voume 40, 2: 318.

91. Yasukawa A, Patel P, Sisung C: Pilot study: investigating the effects of Kinesio Taping in an acute pediatric rehabilitation setting. Am J OccupTher. 2006 Jan-Feb;60(1):104-10.

92. Yin-Hsin Hsu, Wen-Yin Chen, Hsiu-Chen Lin, Wendy T.J. Wang, Yi-Fen Shih: The effects of taping on scapular kinematics and muscle performance in baseball players with shoulder impingement syndrome. J of Electromyography and Kinesio, December 2009:Vol 19, 6: 1092-1099.

93. Yoshida A, Kahanov L:The effect of kinesio taping on lower trunk range of motions. R sprt med, 2007;15(2):103-12.

www.ingramcontent.com/pod-product-compliance
Lightning Source LLC
Chambersburg PA
CBHW081457170526
45166CB00008B/2466